Table of Contents

Introduction 7

    Surf Turf Nachos 9

    Crispy, Crunchy Baked Gluten Free Fried Chicken 11

    Sweet Potato Ragu on a Bed of Rice 13

    Gluten Free Chicken Almond Stir-Fry 15

    Gluten Free Bacon Casserole 18

    Sesame Chicken Stew 20

    Baked, Double Crunch Shrimp 22

    I.P.G.F Scrambled Egg Bowl 24

    Easy G.F. Chicken Noodles 26

    Chicken Salad Sub and Pitas 28

    Greek Chicken Salad Sub and Pitas 30

    Gluten Free Chicken Nuggets Fajita Salad 32

    3-Bean Fajita Salad 34

    Gluten Free Honey Garlic Turkey Penne 36

    Easy Gluten Free Gravy 38

Easy Flourless Gluten Free Gravy 40

Easy Gluten Free Onion and Herb Gravy Over Roasted Potato's 42

Spicy Tofu Mushroom Soup 44

Gluten Free Stir-Fry Rice 46

Gluten Free Chicken Pizza 48

Gluten Free BBQ Chicken Pizza 50

Gluten Free Pizza crust 52

Chicken Chow Mein 54

Sweet Smoky Chicken Kabobs 56

Burger Bake 58

Artic Ranch Fajita Bowl 60

Cauli-Stuffed Peppers 62

G.F. Po Boy 64

Crispy, Baked Gluten Free Fish Sticks 66

Quick Protein Noodles 68

Easy G.F. Eggroll Wrappers 70

Cabbage Eggrolls 72

Cauliflower Gnocchi 74

Gluten Free Fun

50 Great Gluten Free Recipes for Kids & Teens + 1 specialty drink + 5 g.f. desserts!

BY

Julia Chiles

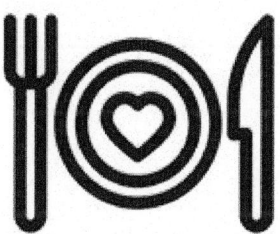

Copyright 2020 - Julia Chiles

License Notes

No part of this Book can be reproduced in any form or by any means including print, electronic, scanning or photocopying unless prior permission is granted by the author.

All ideas, suggestions and guidelines mentioned here are written for informative purposes. While the author has taken every possible step to ensure accuracy, all readers are advised to follow information at their own risk. The author cannot be held responsible for personal and/or commercial damages in case of misinterpreting and misunderstanding any part of this Book

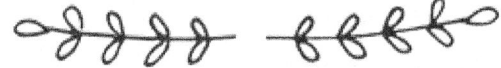

Italiano Chicken with Faux Fried Onion Rings 76

Sweet Heat Fish Sticks 78

Spirals in a Dairy-Free Sauce 80

Baked Chicken Tenders 82

G.F. Mediterranean Quinoa Salad 84

Broiled Shrimp 86

G.F. Baked Chicken Nuggets Cauli-Chips 88

Chickpea Chicken Tenders Broccoli Tots 90

Apple-Cinnamon Pork Chops 92

Sweet Tots 94

Air Fryer Sweet Tots 96

Veggie Sliders 98

Red Pepper and Feta Greek Gluten Free Pizza 100

BBQ Cauliflower Turkey Pizza 102

2-Flour G.F. Pizza crust 104

One Pot G.F. Andouille 106

G.F. Apple Pie French Toast 108

Gluten Dairy-Free Latte 110

Gluten Free Treats 112

    G.F. No-Bake Granola Bites 113

    Bananas and Berries 115

    Easy Gluten Free Nutella Brownies 117

    Peanut Butter Brownies 119

    G.F. Mini Mallow Toffee Brownies 121

    G.F. Chocolate Bread 123

Author's Afterthoughts 125

Introduction

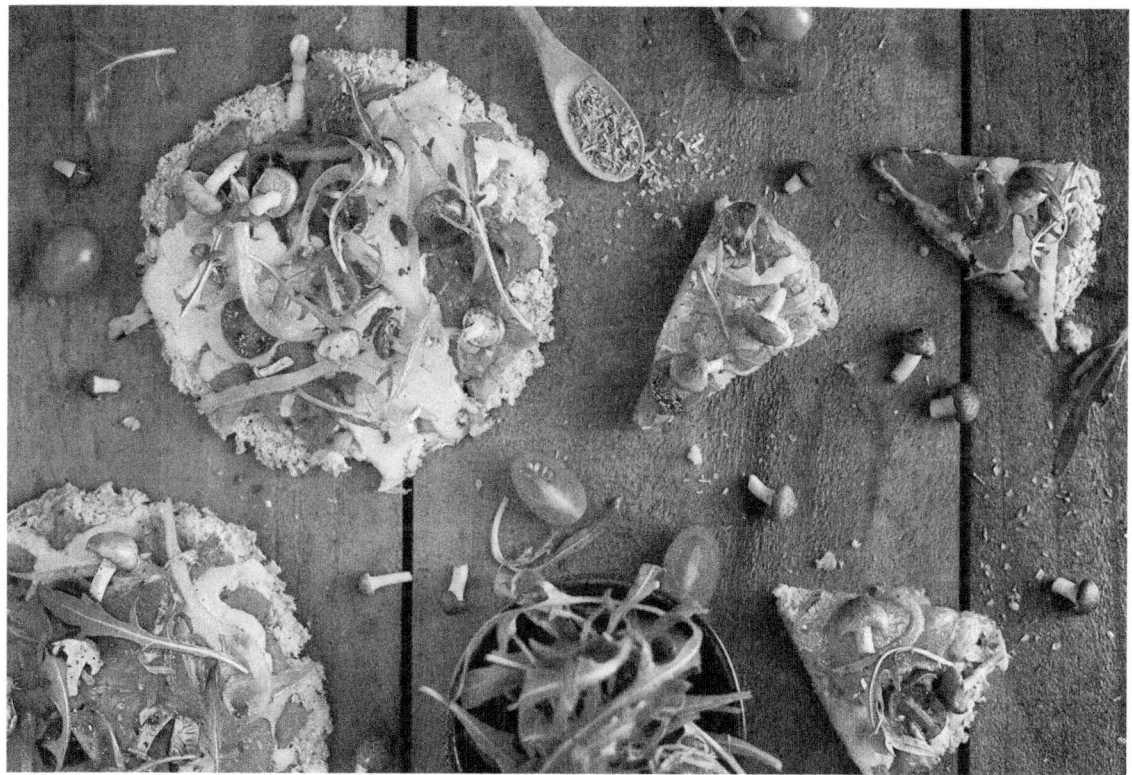

We all know how hard it is to find good gluten free food, but what if you are a kid? The parent of a young gluten free food critic? Or the bored foodie? Gluten Free Fun: 50 Great Gluten Free Recipes for Kids Teens + 1 specialty drink + 5 g.f. desserts! is here to help the culinary challenged!

Gluten Free Fun: 50 Great Gluten Free Recipes for Kids Teen Teens + 1 specialty drink + 5 g.f. desserts! has something for all gluten free pallets 4-16! Crispy, crunchy, double-fried chicken, shrimp, eggrolls, and wrappers. Hearty vegan and vegetarian casseroles, burgers, and soups, comfort foods, stir-fry's, pizza, and much more!

Change the way you eat forever. Give that bland food a g.f. kick and get the most out of your food!

Some Things to Know....

- g.f. - gluten free
- g.f.a.p. - gluten free all-purpose flour
- tsp - teaspoon
- Tbsp - tablespoon
- I.P - Instant Pot

Surf Turf Nachos

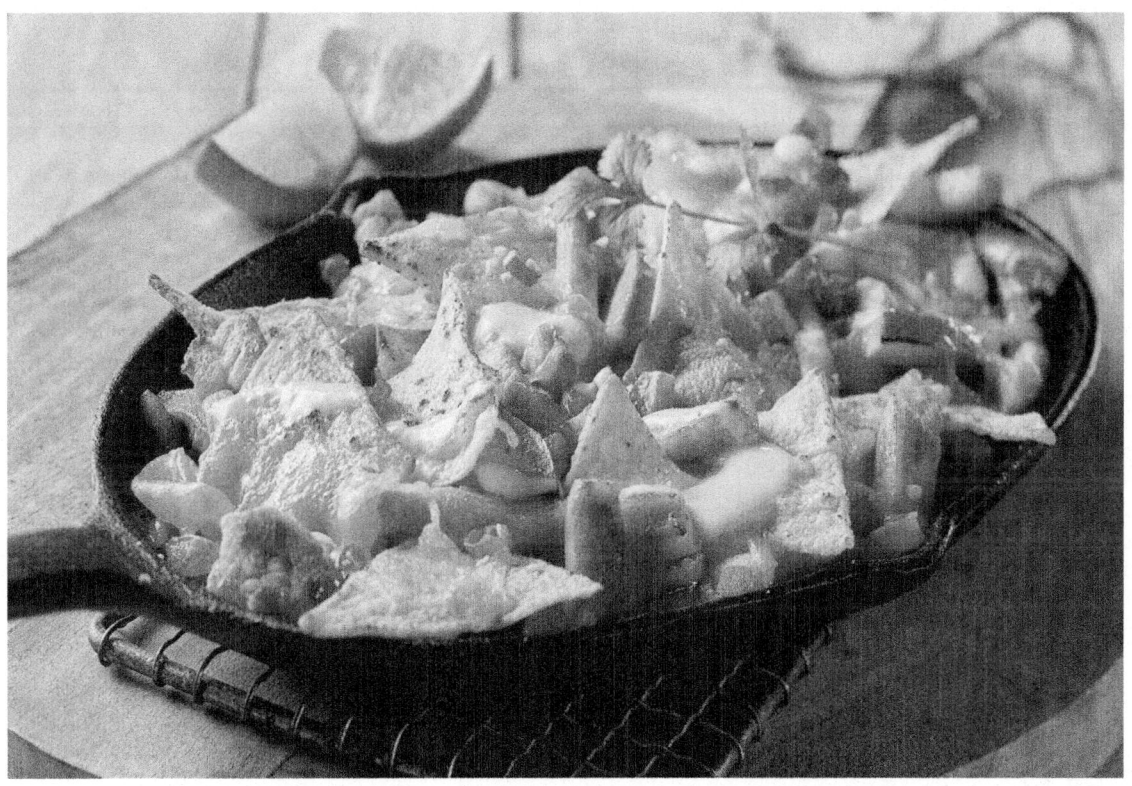

Great way to "sneak" nutrients into kids!! Makes 1 servings.

Ingredients:

- 2-3 cups corn tortilla chips
- ¼-1/3 cup shrimp
- ½ cup ground beef, browned and drained
- ½ tsp chili powder
- 1/3 tsp turmeric
- ½ Tbsp olive oil or coconut oil
- ½ Tbsp butter
- ½ tsp chopped garlic (optional)
- 2 Tbsp mild salsa
- 1/3-1/2 cup shredded cheddar

Directions:

In pot over high heat, mix salsa into browning ground beef.

Transfer to paper towel drain.

In a skillet over medium-high heat melt butter into oil.

Stir in turmeric, chili powder, garlic.

Add shrimp and sauté 30 seconds.

Transfer to a paper towel and drain.

Spread tortilla chips on pan and top with cheese, shrimp, and burger.

Broil 1-2 minutes or until cheese melts.

Crispy, Crunchy Baked Gluten Free Fried Chicken

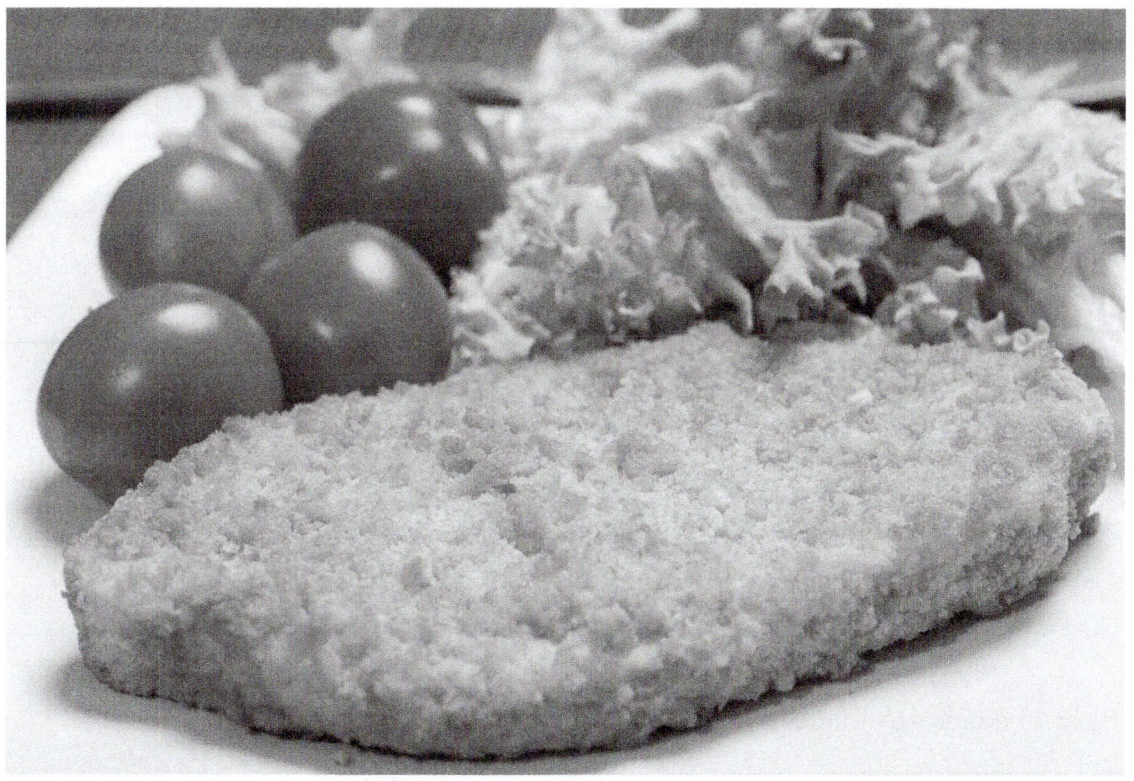

Use a good 1 to 1 g.f.a.p flour!! Makes 2 servings.

Ingredients:

- Olive oil spray
- 2 chicken breasts/filets
- 1 cup gluten free all-purpose flour
- ½ cup gluten free breadcrumbs

Directions:

Preheat oven to 425 and prepare a pan.

Thaw chicken.

Coat both sides with flour and shake off excess.

Coat both sides with g.f breadcrumbs and shake off excess.

Bake 45 minutes to 1 hr. depending on the thickness.

CDC guidelines state it is done at an internal temp of 165.

Sweet Potato Ragu on a Bed of Rice

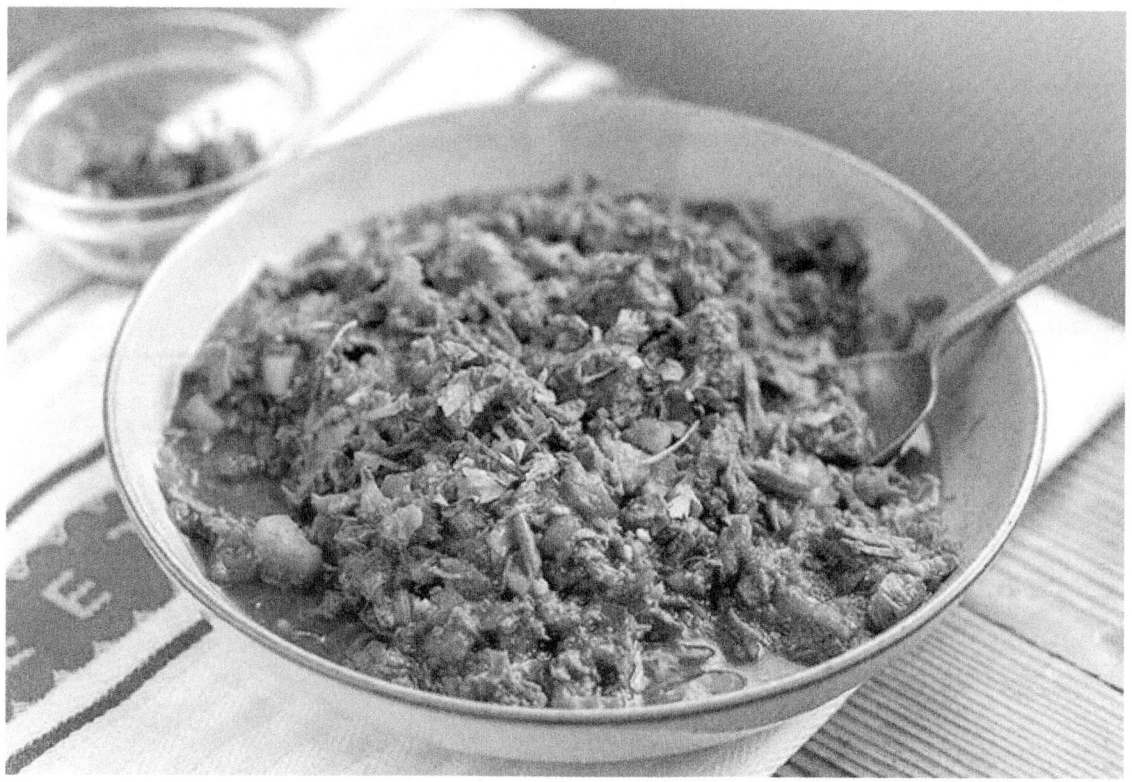

For the older, more discriminating tastes! Makes 1 serving.

Ingredients:

- 1 cup rice
- 1 cup ground beef, browned and drained
- 1 chopped medium sweet potato
- ½ tablespoon crushed walnuts or silvered almonds
- 1/2 cup diced mushrooms
- ½ tablespoon diced thyme
- ½ tablespoon diced oregano
- Shredded cheddar cheese for topping

Directions:

Fix rice into a bed on plate.

Sauté nuts, mushrooms, thyme, oregano 30-45 seconds.

Add in sweet potato and ground beef.

Warm through.

Spoon on top of rice.

Gluten Free Chicken Almond Stir-Fry

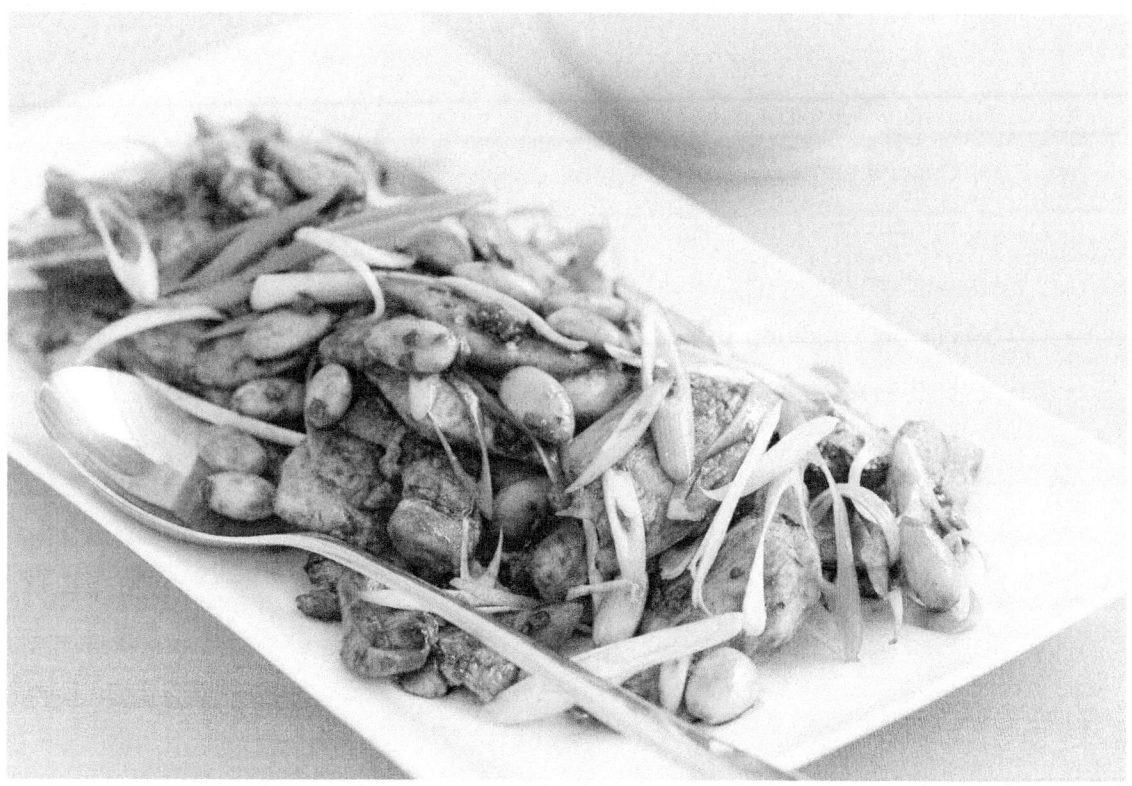

Also great with ground turkey! Makes 1 servings.

Ingredients:

- 2 Tbsp olive oil
- 1/3 tsp rice vinegar
- ½ Tbsp diced onion
- ½ tsp minced garlic
- 1-2 drops chili oil (optional)
- ½ tsp chicken bouillon granules
- 1/2-piece ginger chopped
- 1 Tbsp slivered almonds
- ¼ cup diced or shredded chicken
- 1/2 cup cooked jasmine rice

Directions:

Preheat oven to 350 and prepare 8x8 pan.

Warm skillet over high heat and toast almonds until fragrant.

In small bowl whisk together oil, vinegar, onion, garlic, chili oil, bouillon granules and ginger.

Transfer almonds to paper towel.

Pour oil mixture in skillet.

Let chicken pieces sit 2 minutes before moving. They should be a nice golden brown, flip, repeat.

Pour in cooked rice and toss.

Top with almonds.

Gluten Free Bacon Casserole

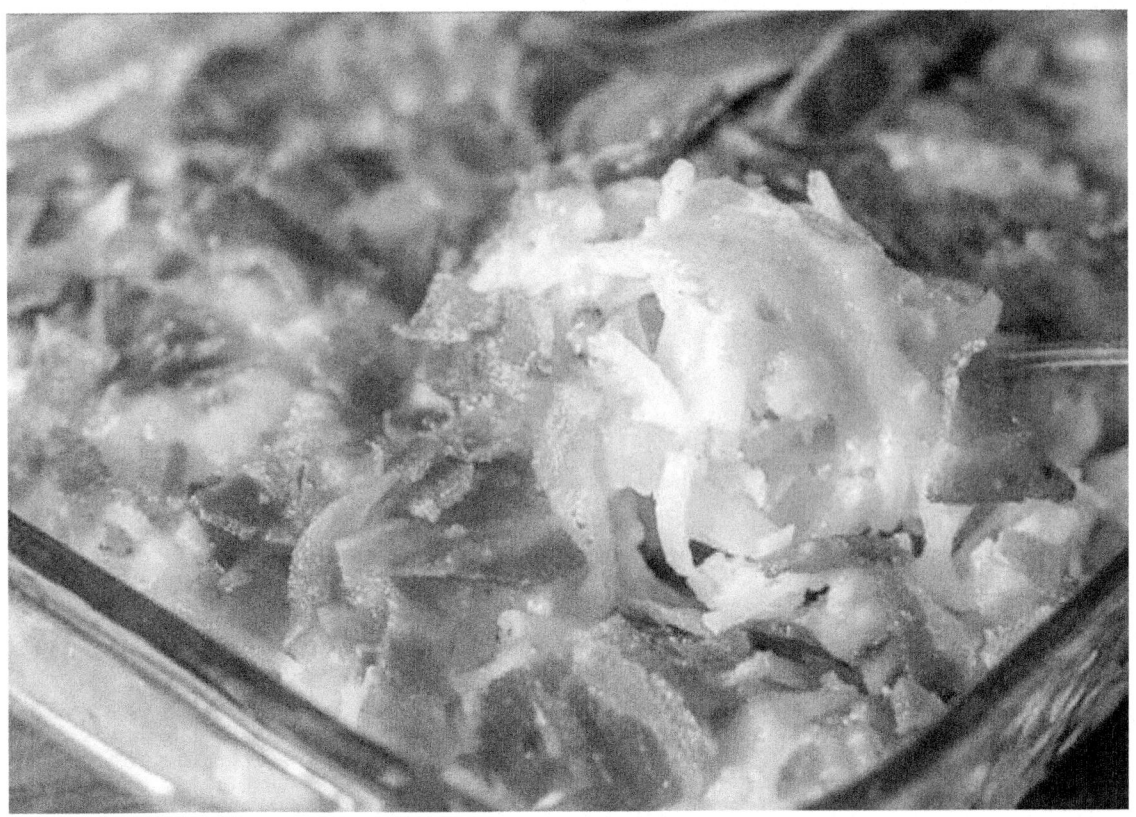

Great as a casserole! Makes 2 servings.

Ingredients:

- 1/2 cup turkey bacon, chopped
- 12/3 cup diced onion
- 2 crushed cloves of garlic
- 4 cups of chopped cabbage
- 1/4 cup toasted almond slivers
- 1/3 cup multicolored bell peppers, diced
- 1/3 cup grated parmesan
- Olive oil for drizzling

Directions:

In skillet warmed over medium heat and oil sauté pancetta, onions, garlic 45 seconds – 1 minute.

Add in almond slivers, and diced bell peppers.

Cover bottom of 8x8 pan with cabbage, layer with 1/3 cup pancetta mix and some cheese. Repeat.

Drizzle with olive oil.

Bake 25-30 minutes.

Sesame Chicken Stew

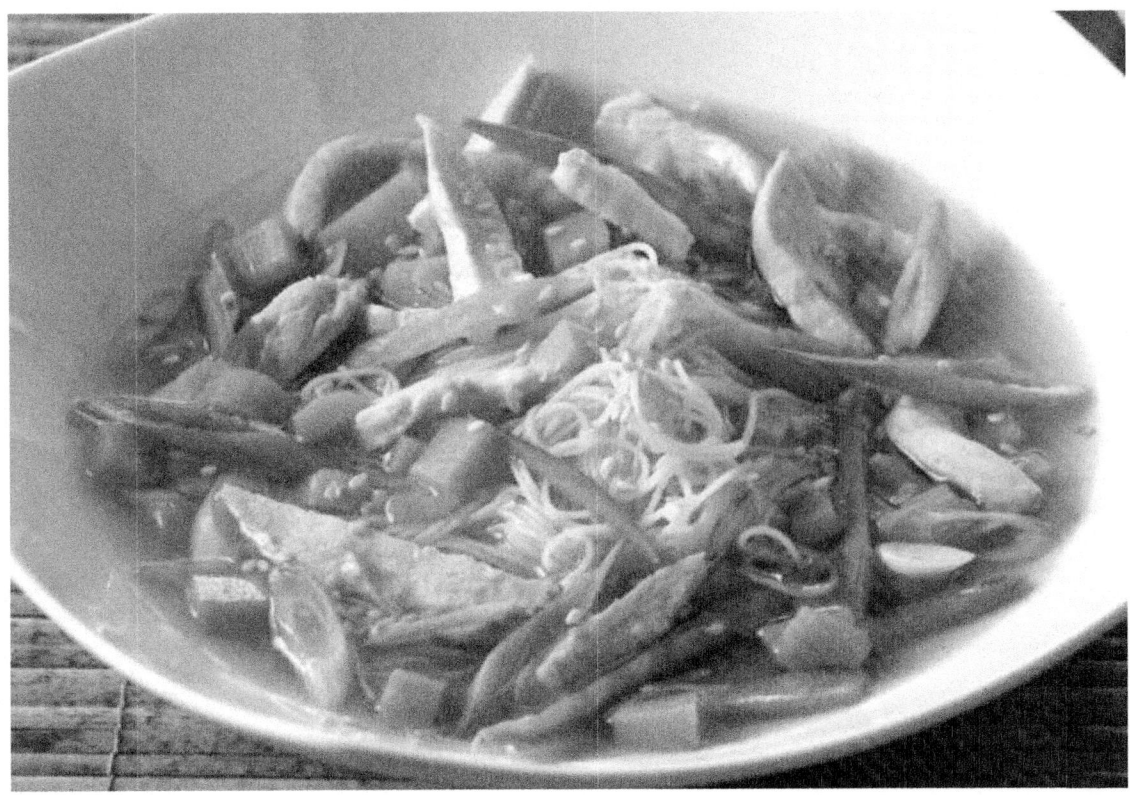

Great pressure cooker meal! Makes 2 servings.

Ingredients:

- 1/2 teaspoon sesame oil
- ½ tsp onion powder
- ½ cup ground chicken
- 1 tsp garlic, minced
- 1/4 cup matchstick carrots
- ½ Tbsp tomato paste
- 1 cup worth rice noodles
- ½ teaspoon diced oregano
- 1/3 cup vegetable or beef stock
- 1 tsp cornstarch

Directions:

In pot combine sesame oil, onion powder, chicken, matchstick carrots, tomato paste, noodles, oregano, stock.

Stir in cornstarch.

Bring to a boil, reduce heat, cover, and let simmer 15-20 minutes.

Baked, Double Crunch Shrimp

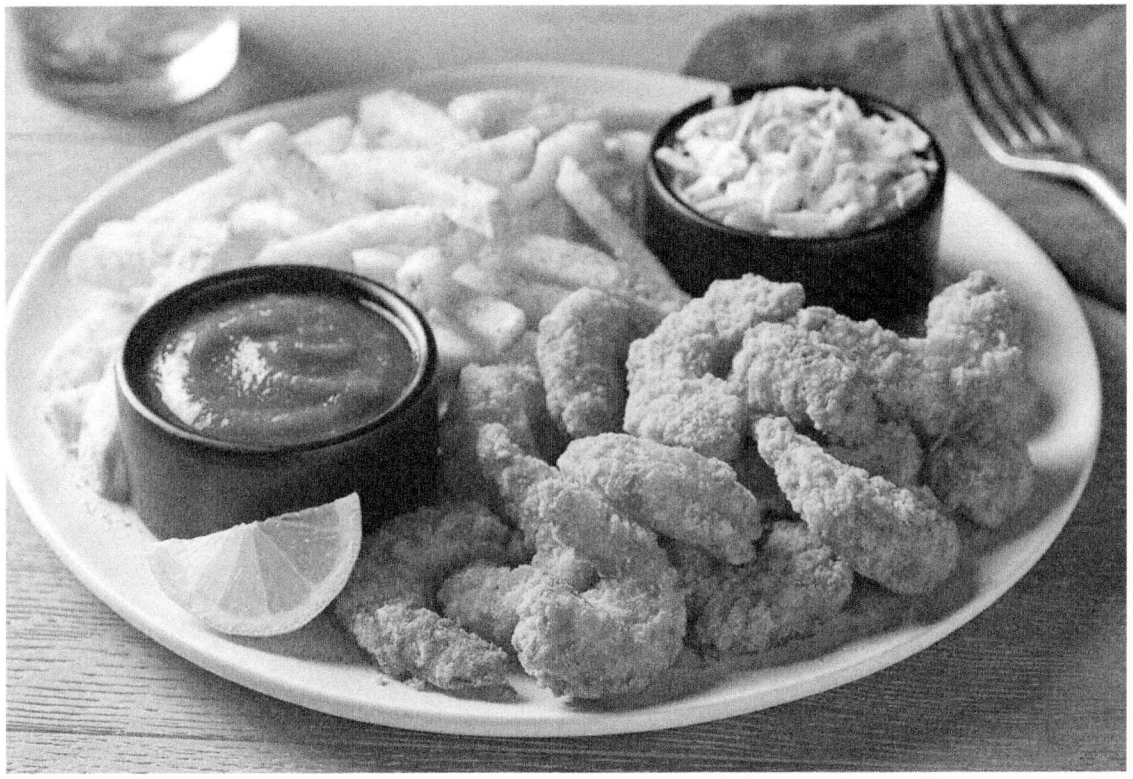

Use your favorite spices in the flour! Makes 2 servings.

Ingredients:

- 8-10 medium shrimp, peeled and deveined
- 1/2 tablespoon butter
- ½ cup all-purpose gluten free flour
- 1 cup gluten free all-purpose flour
- 1 teaspoon garlic powder with parsley
- 1 teaspoon paprika
- Preheat oven to 400 and prepare baking sheet.

Directions:

Mix flour, garlic powder, and paprika together.

Coat shrimp with a.p.g.f. flour, shake off excess.

Coat shrimp in g.f. breadcrumbs, shake off the excess.

Spread out on pan.

Cook 20-30 minutes

I.P.G.F Scrambled Egg Bowl

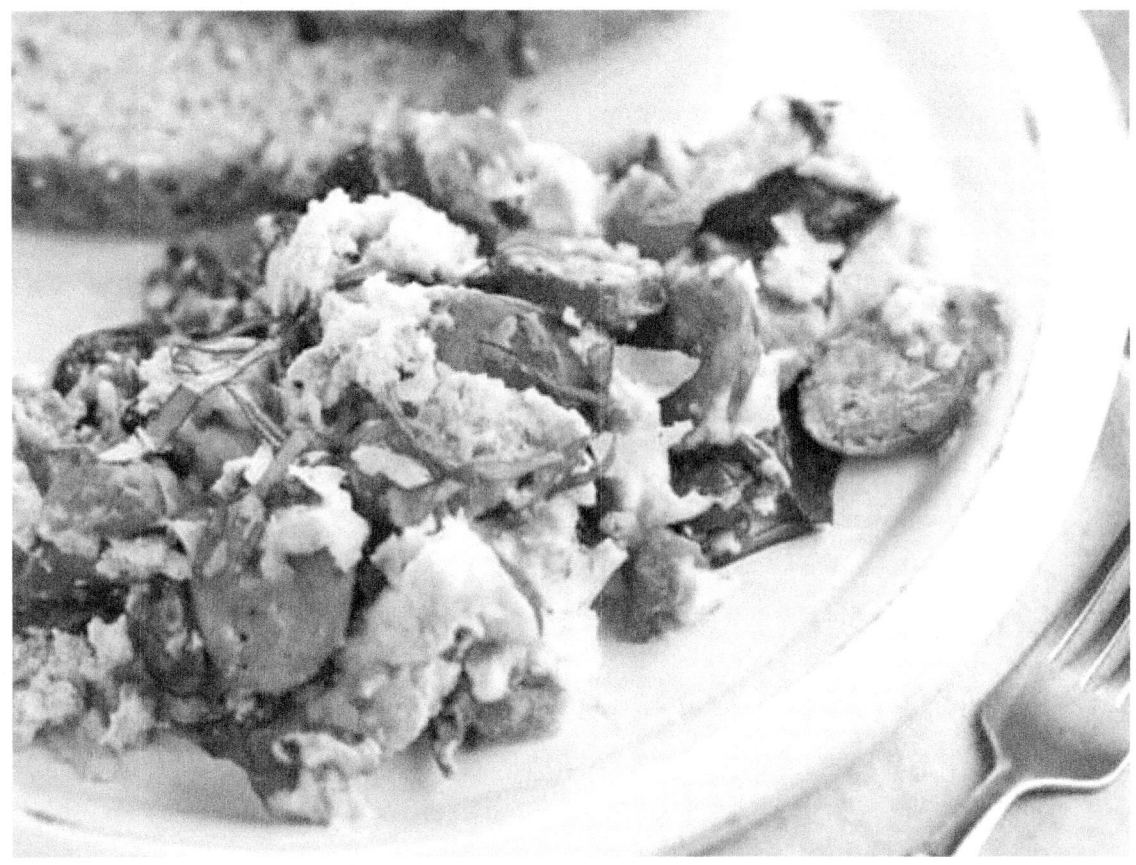

Let the instant pot do breakfast! Makes 2 bowls.

Ingredients:

- Coconut or avocado oil
- 4 eggs, beaten
- 1 cup baby spinach or kale
- ½ Tbsp tomato paste
- 2 scallions, thinly sliced
- 1 teaspoon turmeric
- ½ tsp Italian seasoning

Directions:

In skillet warmed over medium high heat whisk together oil, beaten eggs, turmeric, and paste.

Add in spinach and scallions.

Scramble and divide between two bowls

Easy G.F. Chicken Noodles

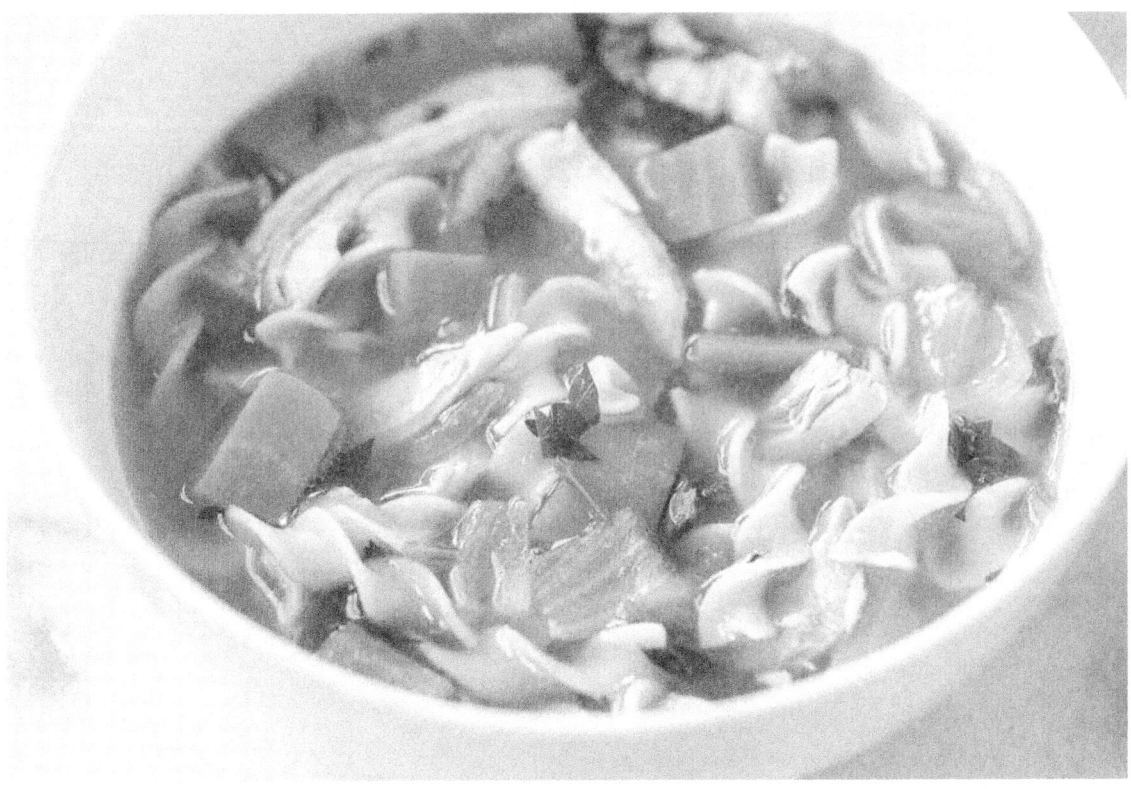

Perfect for lean proteins! Makes 2 servings.

Ingredients:

- ½ cup leftover chicken or ½ cup ground chicken browned and drained
- 1/4 cup diced onions
- 1 teaspoon minced garlic
- 1/2 teaspoon pepper
- ½ cup matchstick carrots
- water
- 1 package lemongrass and chili rice noodles (such as Thai Kitchen)

Directions:

In microwave safe dish add onions, garlic, pepper, matchstick carrots, vegetable broth, rice noodles, and quantity of water as directed.

Cook on high heat 3-4 minutes.

Meanwhile, scramble egg and pour into noodles and bok choy.

Chicken Salad Sub and Pitas

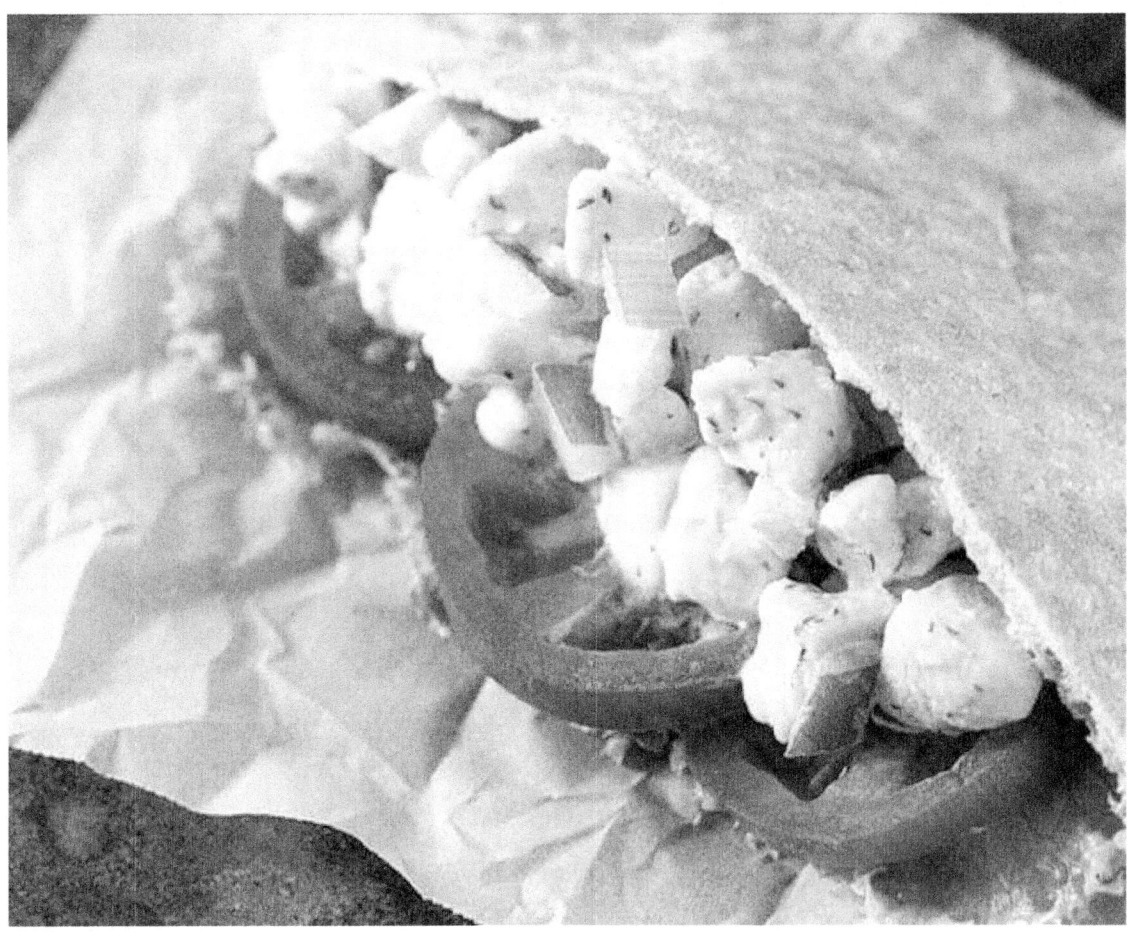

Try using fresh herbs. Makes 2 servings.

Ingredients:

- ½ tsp Italian seasoning
- 1 clove garlic, minced
- ½ cup low fat mayo
- 1/3 cup chunked chicken
- ¼ cup lettuce
- 4 sliced cherry tomatoes
- 1 g.f. sub bun
- 10 pita chips
- 1 tub hummus

Directions:

Mix together seasoning, garlic, mayo, chicken.

Cover and chill in refrigerator 10 minutes.

Spoon evenly into bun.

Top with tomatoes and lettuce.

Place pitas around sub with tub of hummus.

Greek Chicken Salad Sub and Pitas

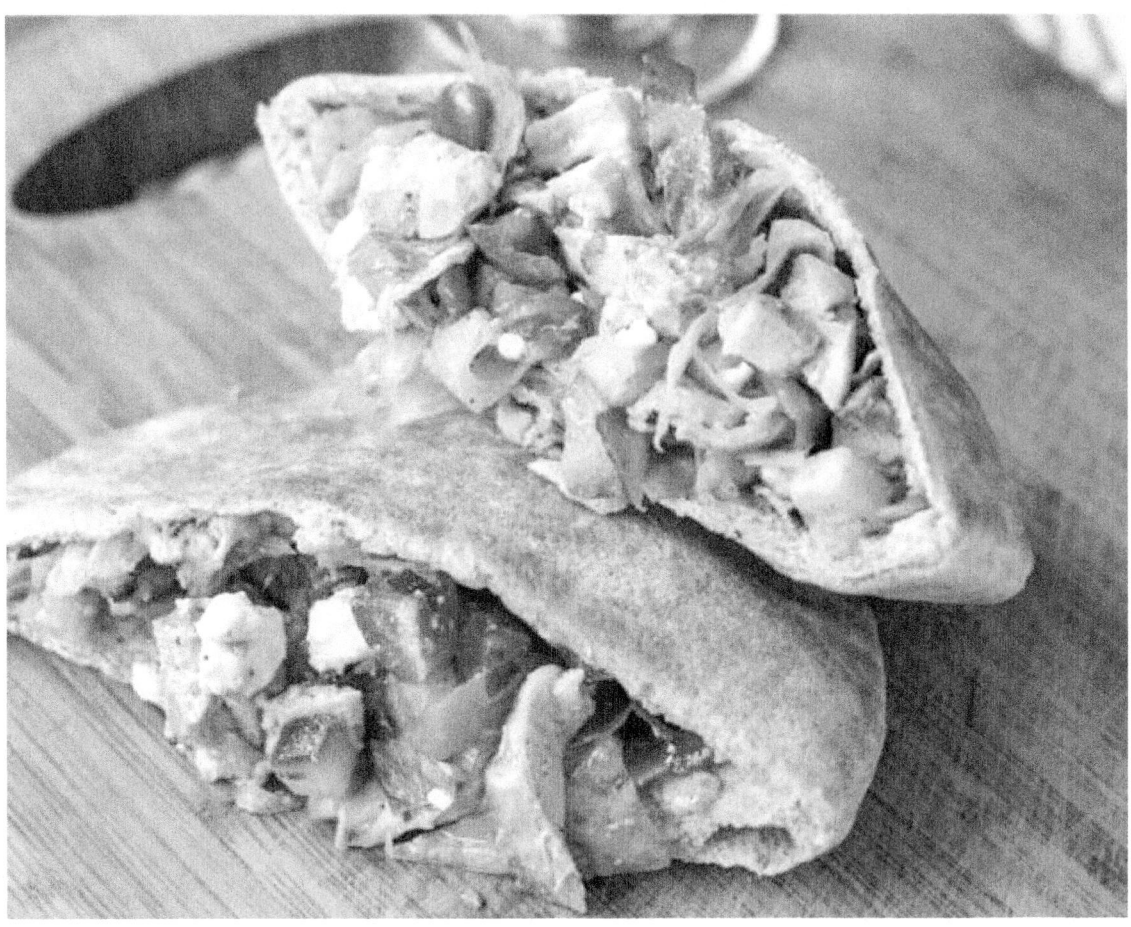

Try adding lemon peel! Makes 1 serving

Ingredients:

- ½ tsp Greek seasoning
- 2-3 cloves garlic, minced
- ½ cup low fat mayo
- 1/3 cup chunked chicken
- ¼ cup lettuce
- 4 sliced cherry tomatoes
- 1 g.f. sub bun
- 10 pita chips
- 1 tub hummus

Directions:

Mix together seasoning, garlic, mayo, chicken.

Cover and chill in refrigerator 10 minutes.

Spoon evenly into bun.

Top with tomatoes and lettuce.

Place pitas around sub with tub of hummus.

Gluten Free Chicken Nuggets Fajita Salad

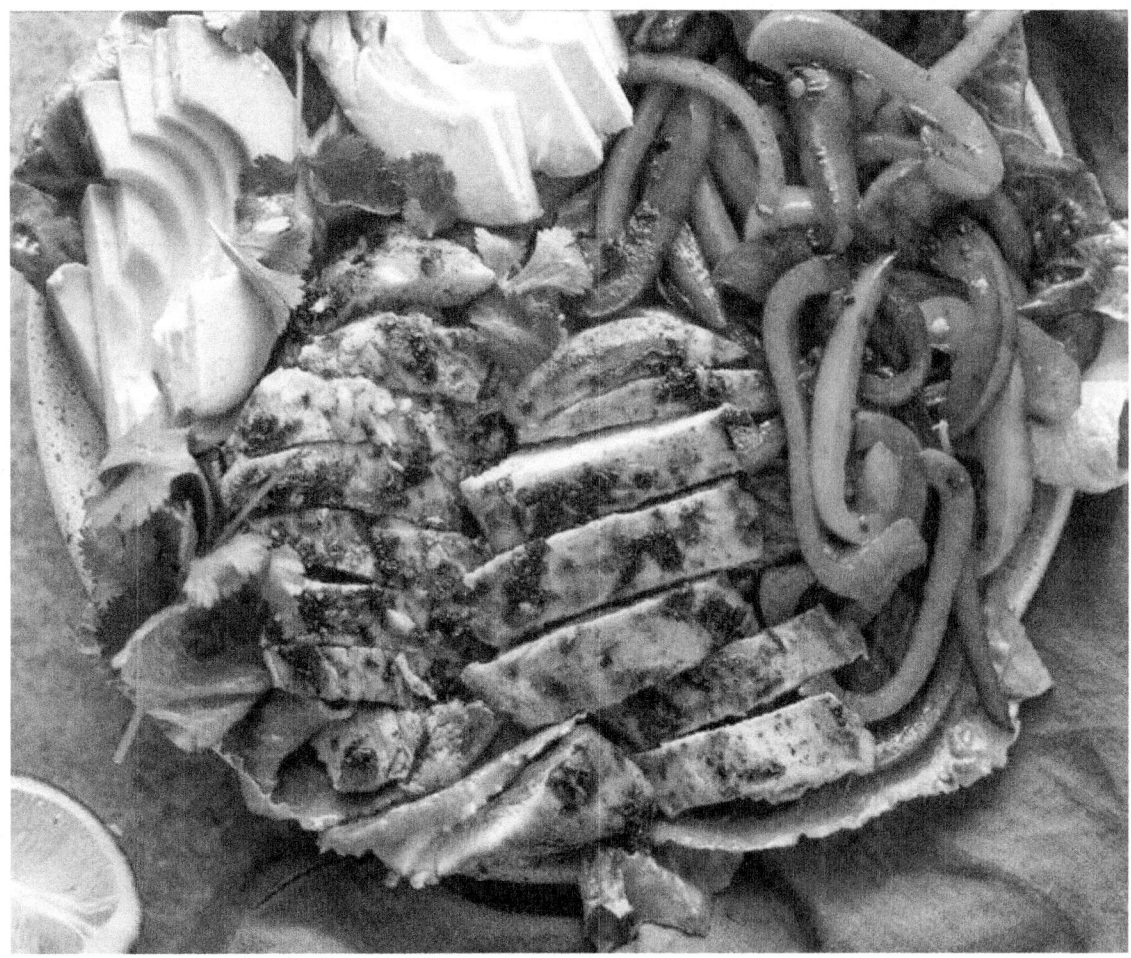

Also, great with steak! Makes 2 servings.

Ingredients:

- 1 boneless, skinless chicken breast cut to nugget sizes and cooked as directed by Crispy, Crunchy, Baked Fried Chicken recipe
- 1 bell pepper, julienned
- 1 cup shredded lettuce
- 2-3 diced fire roasted tomatoes, no-salt added
- 1 can organic blackbeans, washed (optional)
- ½ tablespoon lime juice
- 1 tablespoon chili powder
- 1 teaspoon ground cumin
- 1 teaspoon brown sugar
- 1/4 teaspoon cayenne pepper
- 1 corn tortilla bowl
- Salsa for topping (optional)
- Sour cream for topping (optional)

Directions:

Cook and prepare nuggets as described in Crispy, Crunchy Baked Fried Chicken

In a small bowl combine olive oil, lime juice, chili powder, ground cumin, coriander, brown sugar, cayenne pepper, bell peppers rings, cover and chill in fridge

In separate container combine lettuce, tomatoes, and blackbeans and let chill in refrigerator.

Pour over oil mixture over salad and toss.

Pour into tortilla bowl and top as desired.

3-Bean Fajita Salad

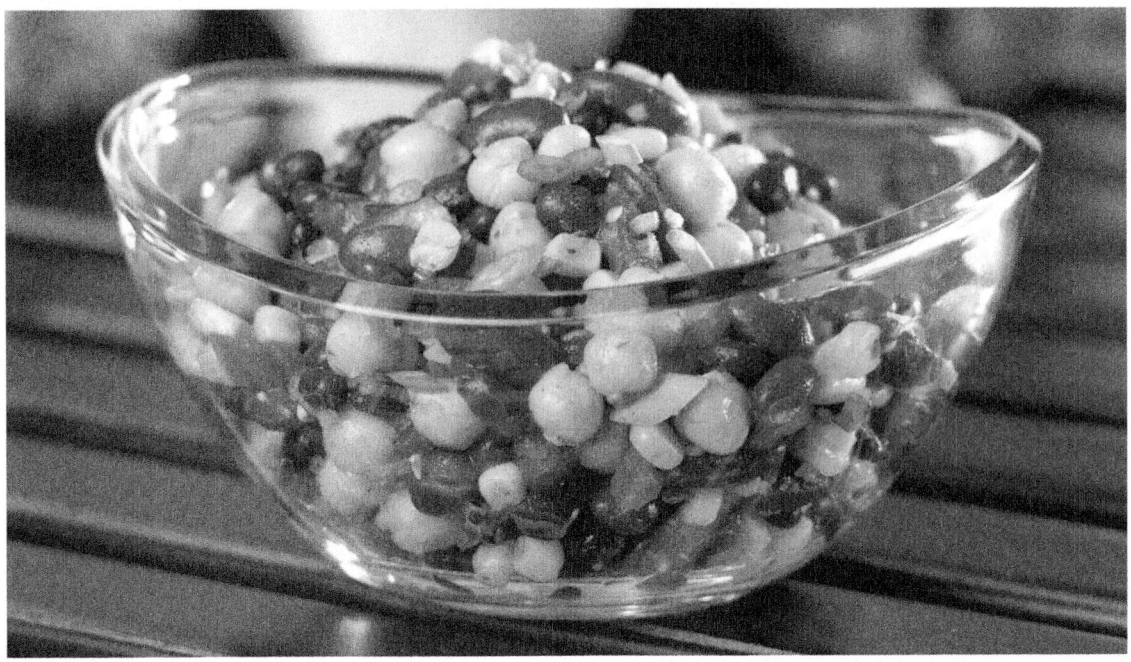

Try in different beans! Makes 2 servings.

Ingredients:

- 1/2 cup low sodium garbanzo beans, washed and drained
- ½ can low sodium red kidney beans, washed and drained
- ½ cab pinto beans, washed and drained
- 1 bell pepper, julienned
- 1/3 cup shredded lettuce, washed and drained
- 1/3 diced tomatoes
- ½ tablespoon lime juice
- 1 tablespoons chili powder
- 1 teaspoon ground cumin
- 1/4 teaspoon cayenne pepper
- 1 corn tortilla bowl

Directions:

Combine lettuce, tomatoes and let chill in fridge.

In skillet combine beans, lime juice, chili powder, ground cumin, coriander, brown sugar, cayenne pepper.

Sauté chicken and peppers in skillet over olive oil 1-2 minutes.

Pour over lettuce, tomatoes and top as desired.

Gluten Free Honey Garlic Turkey Penne

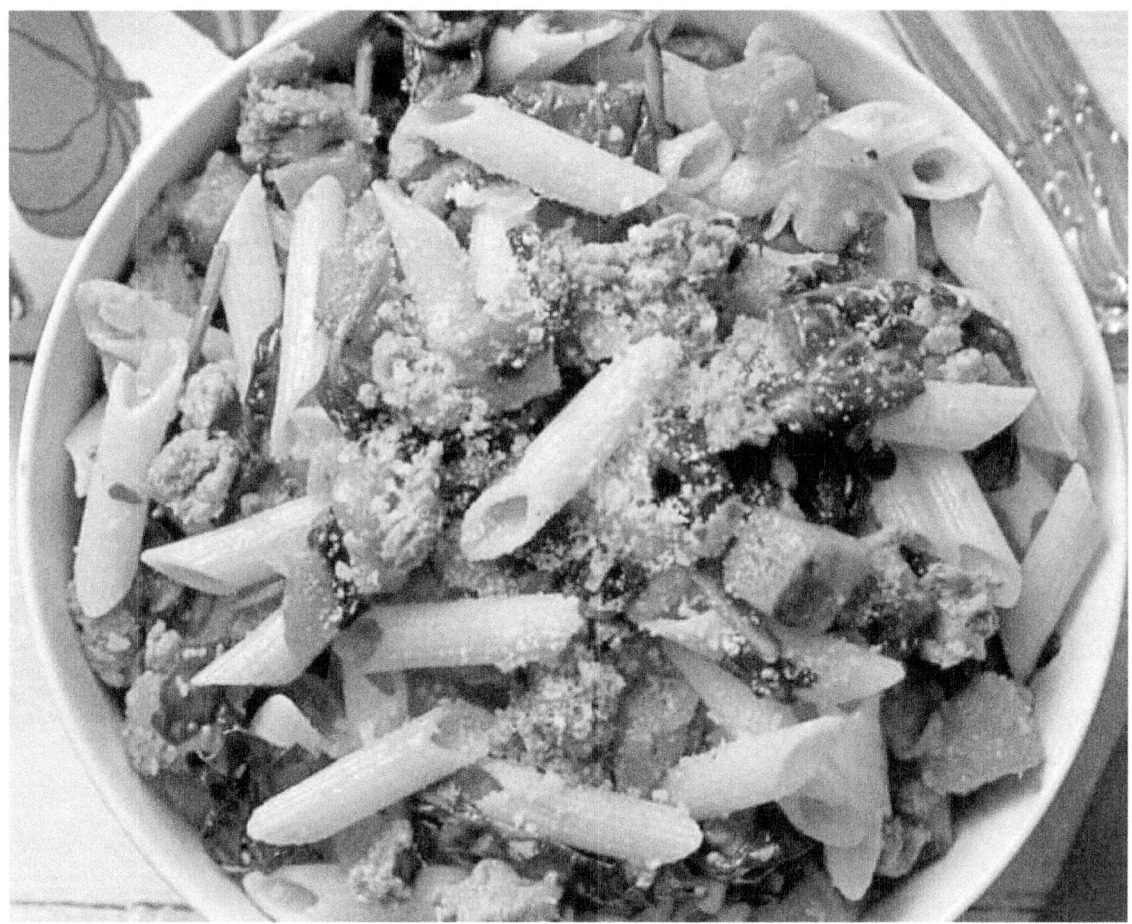

Great for disguising vegetables! Makes 1 servings.

Ingredients:

- 1 cup ground turkey
- 1 Tbsp olive oil (use coconut oil for a change of flavor)
- ½ Tbsp pepper
- 1/3 cup bell pepper, diced (optional)
- 1 tsp garlic, minced or grated
- 2 teaspoons organic honey
- 1 teaspoon walnuts
- 1 Tbsp-1/4 cup spinach diced
- ½ Tbsp diced parsley, diced
- 1/3 cup g.f. penne pasta, cooked al dente and drained- DO NOT RINSE

Directions:

In a skillet warmed over high heat brown turkey.

Transfer to paper towel.

To skillet add oil, pepper, diced bell peppers, garlic, spinach, and walnuts. And sauté 25-30 seconds.

Toss in turkey and warm through.

Toss in penne.

Easy Gluten Free Gravy

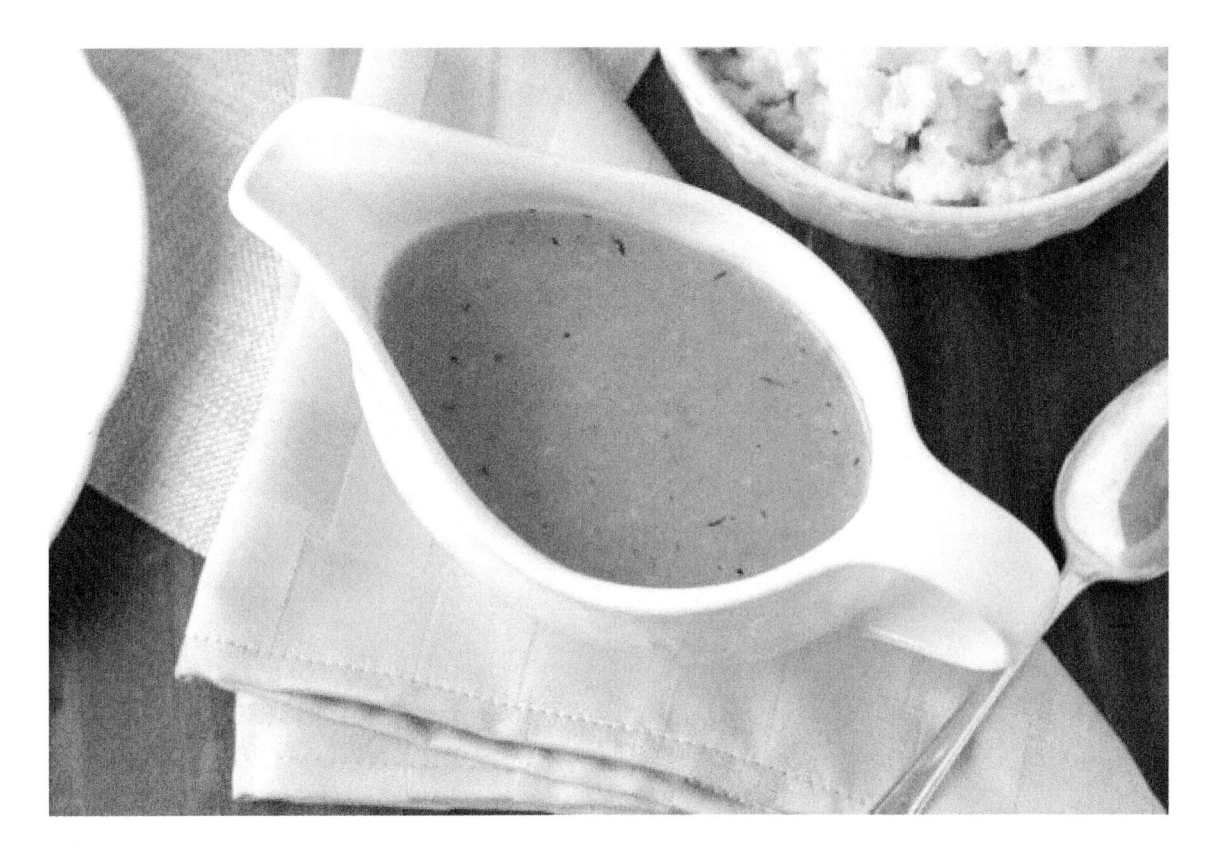

For this recipe, a 1-1 ratio g.f.a.p. flour with xanthan gum works! Makes 4-5 servings.

Ingredients:

- ¼ cup + ½ Tbsp g.f. flour
- 2 ½ cup broth/stock or warm turkey drippings
- 3-4 Tbsp butter

Directions:

When using g.f. flour with xanthan gum or starches, add these ingredients to the cold mixture or it will clump! Always use cold ingredients and put everything in a pot before turning on the burner. Any butter (regular, dairy-free, clarified, etc.) or broth/stock/bouillon cubes work. Bring turkey drippings to room temp before using. To thicken gravy, add g.f. flour to 2-3 Tbsp cold broth/stock or room temp turkey drippings then mix into the main gravy supply.

Easy Flourless Gluten Free Gravy

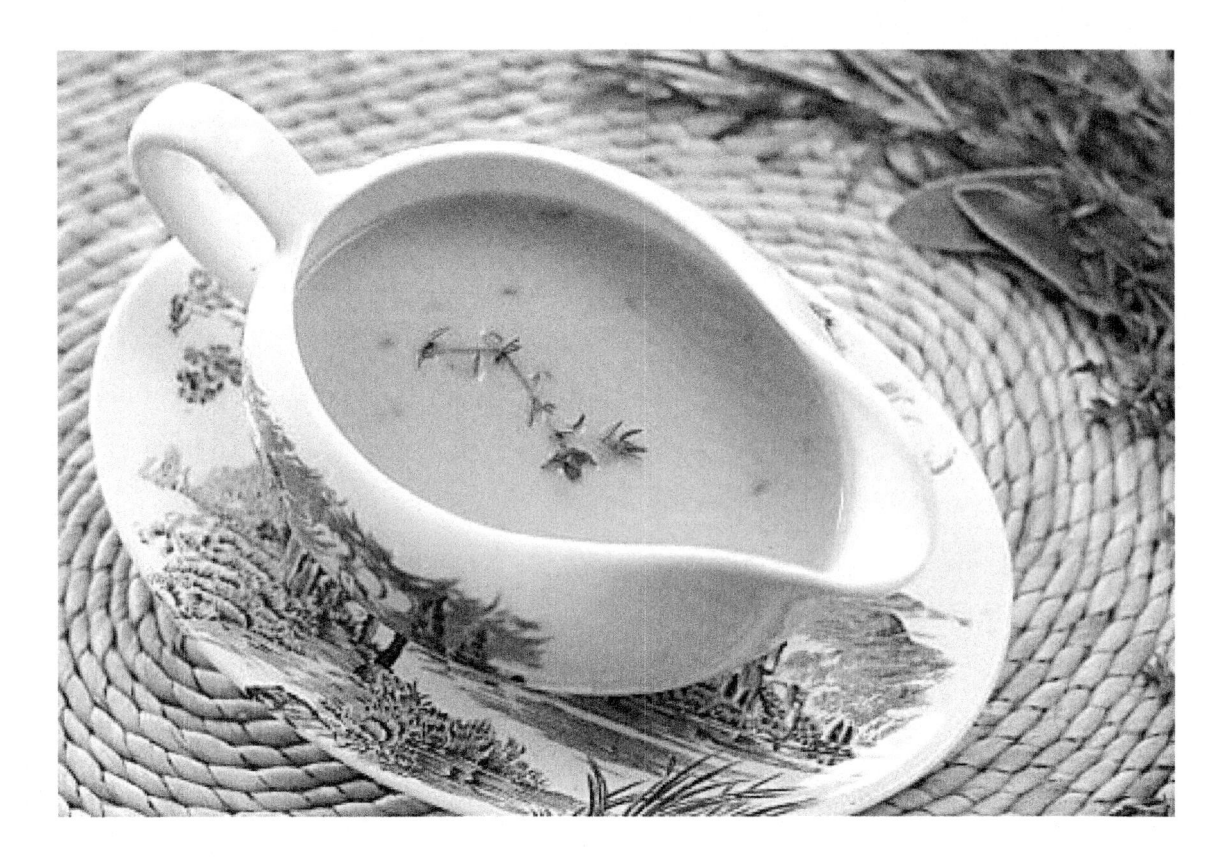

Anybody can do this! Makes 4-5 servings.

Ingredients:

- ¼ cup +1 tsp cornstarch
- 2 ½ cup broth/stock or warm turkey drippings
- 3-4 Tbsp butter

Directions:

When using a flour with xanthan gum or starches, add these ingredients to the cold mixture or it will clump! Always use cold ingredients and put everything in a pot before turning on the burner. Any butter (regular, dairy-free, clarified, etc.) or broth/stock/bouillon cubes work. Bring turkey drippings to room temp before using. To thicken gravy, add g.f. flour to 2-3 Tbsp cold broth/stock or room temp turkey drippings then mix into the main gravy supply.

Easy Gluten Free Onion and Herb Gravy Over Roasted Potato's

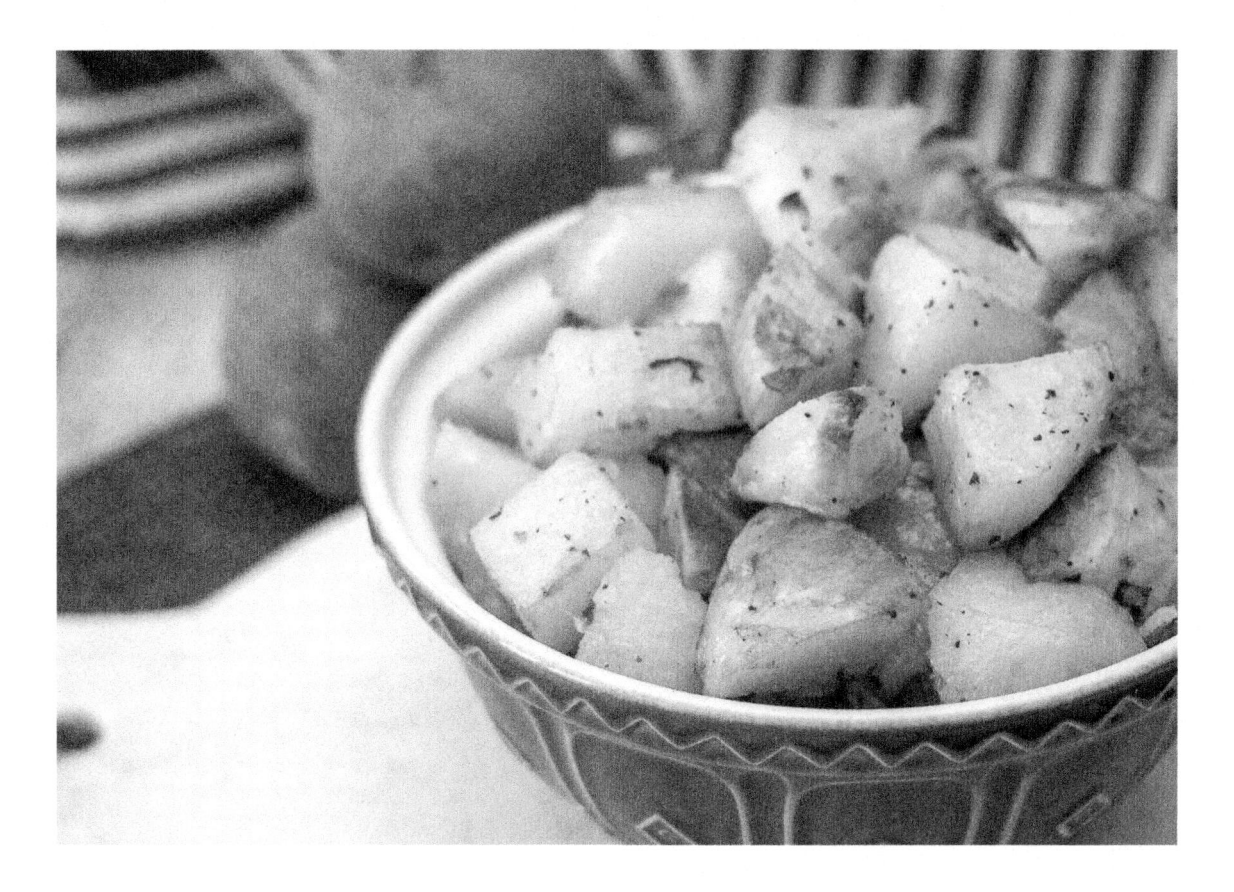

Chia seed powder is full of antioxidants, fiber, and omega-3 Makes 4-6 servings.

Ingredients:

- 15-20 small purple potatoes
- Olive oil for drizzling
- 1/3 cup diced onions
- 2 cup stock or water
- 2-3 Tbsp chia seed powder
- 1 teaspoon finely diced Italian oregano
- 1 teaspoon finely diced rosemary

Directions:

Preheat oven to 400 and line baking sheet with aluminum foil.

Quarter cut potatoes, lay in single layer on sheet and drizzle with olive oil.

Bake 38-42 minutes.

In skillet toast chia seed powder.

Whisk in stock/water, wine, chopped scallions, and diced leeks.

Bring to a boil, cover, reduce heat and simmer 25-30 minutes or until reduced by half. Stir occasionally.

Stir in diced oregano, thyme, and rosemary.

Spicy Tofu Mushroom Soup

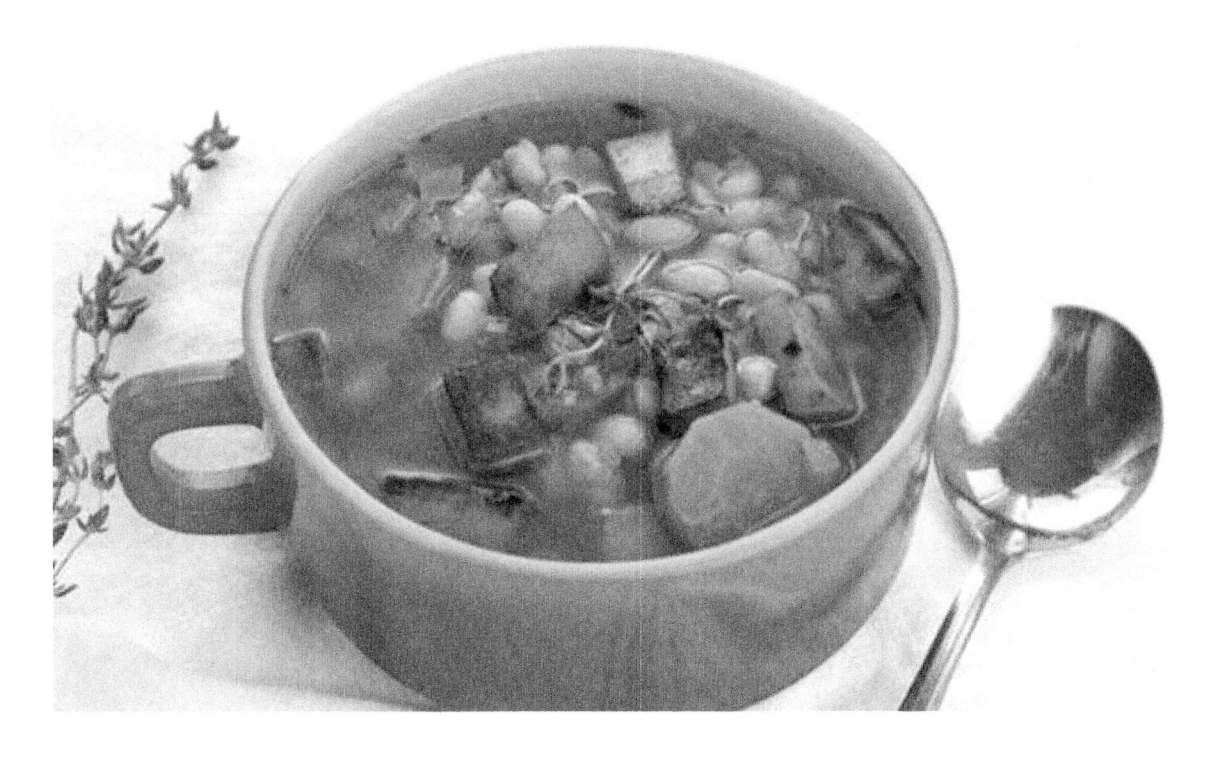

Great vegetarian meal! Makes 2 servings.

Ingredients:

- ½ block firm, silken tofu
- 1 cup shiitake mushrooms, sliced
- 1 teaspoon ground ginger
- 1 teaspoon ground turmeric or paprika
- ¼ tsp five spice powder
- 1/3 tsp oregano
- 1/4 tsp rosemary
- 1/3 cups garbanzo beans, washed and drained
- 2-3 cups beef or vegetable stock

Directions:

In pot combine tofu, mushrooms, ginger, turmeric, five spice powder, oregano, rosemary, beans, stock.

Bring to a boil, cover, reduce heat and let simmer 10-15 minutes.

Gluten Free Stir-Fry Rice

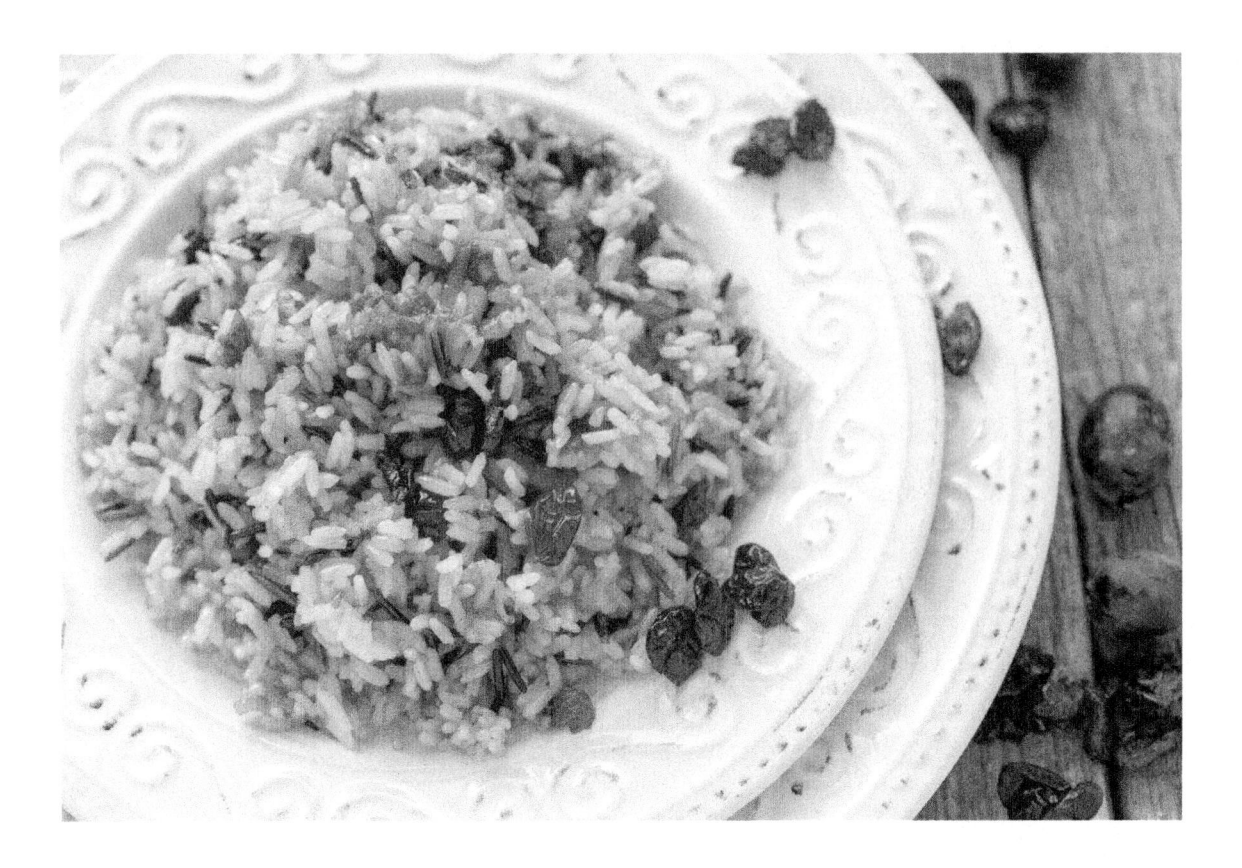

Pomegranates have anti-inflammatory properties! Makes 2 servings.

Ingredients:

- ½ jasmine rice
- ½ Tbsp olive oil or coconut oil
- ¼ cup walnuts
- ¼ cup julienned onions
- ¼ cup dried cranberries or pomegranates
- ¼ cup diced bell peppers

Directions:

In pot combine oil, walnuts, onions, cranberries/pomegranates, and bell peppers.

Sauté 1 minute.

Add in rice and stock.

Bring to boil, reduce heat, cover, let simmer 10-15 minutes.

Gluten Free Chicken Pizza

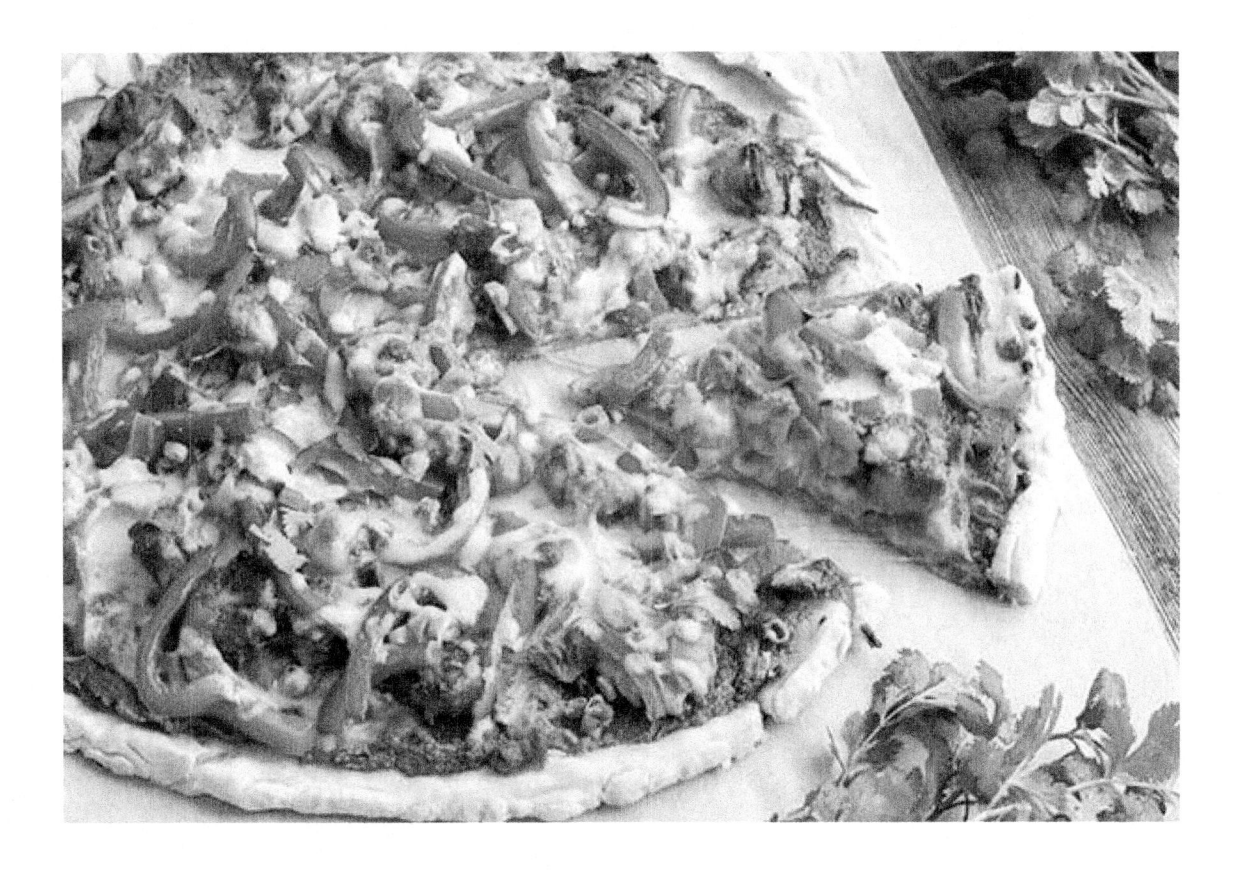

Friends on keto? Here's one for you both!! Makes 1 pizza.

Ingredients:

- 2/3 cup chicken shredded
- ½-1/3 cup crumbled feta cheese
- ½ tsp garlic, minced
- ¼ tsp onion grated or minced
- 2-3 sweet red pepper, chopped- stems and seed removed
- ¼ teaspoon Italian seasoning
- 1 cauliflower pizza crust

Directions:

In blender or food processor add red pepper pieces, Italian seasoning, grated or minced onion and minced garlic. Puree or leave chunky thickens depends on thick you like your sauce.

Spread sauce on cauliflower crust and top with shredded chicken and cheese.

Gluten Free BBQ Chicken Pizza

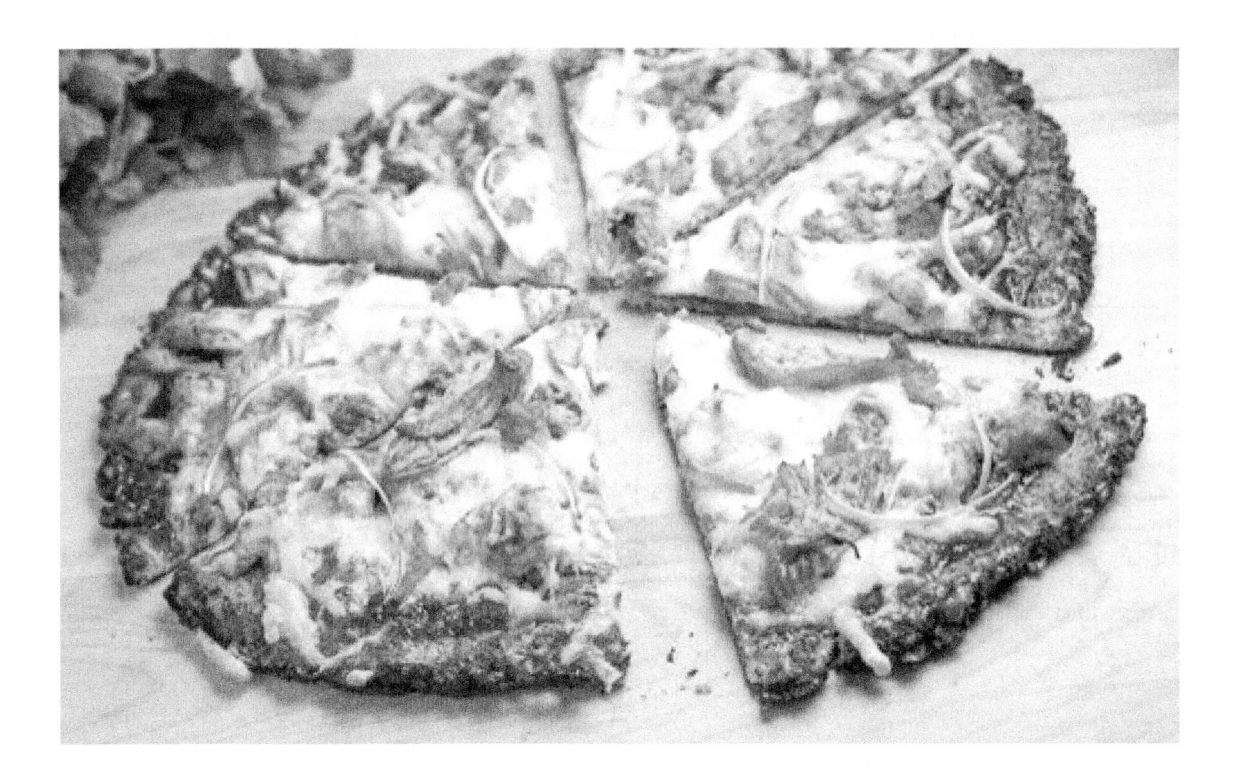

Love! Makes 1 pizza.

Ingredients:

- 2/3 cup BBQ chicken shredded
- ½-1/3 cup crumbled feta cheese
- ½ tsp garlic, minced
- ¼ tsp onion powder or julienned and caramelized
- 2-3 sweet red pepper, chopped- stems and seed removed
- ¼ teaspoon Italian seasoning
- 1 cauliflower pizza crust

Directions:

Mix together BBQ sauce, Italian seasoning, onion powder and minced garlic.

Spread sauce on cauliflower crust and top with shredded chicken and cheese

Gluten Free Pizza crust

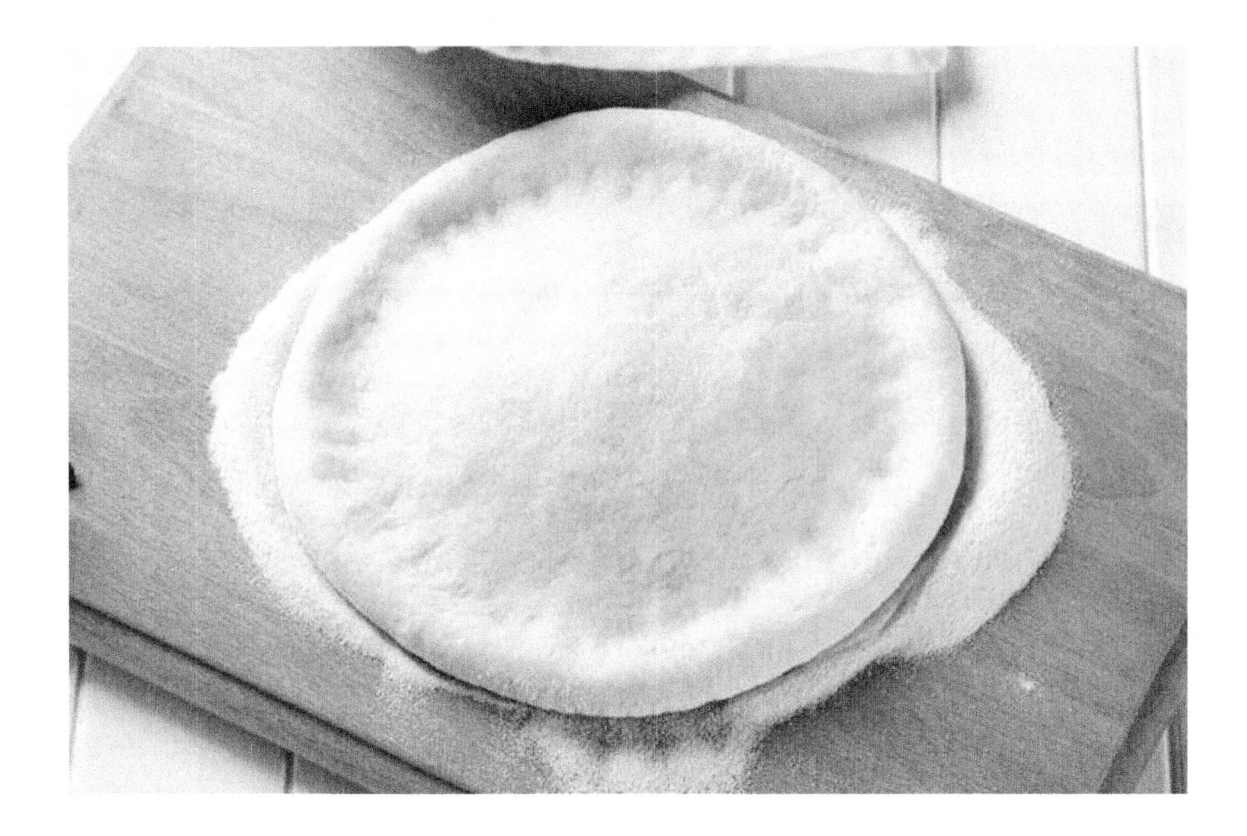

Great for Margarita Pizza's! Makes 1 12-14-inch pizza crust, 50 grams of carbs

Ingredients:

- ¾ cup tapioca flour
- 1/3 cup coconut flour
- 1/2 cup olive oil
- 1/2 cup warm water
- 1 large egg

Directions:

Preheat oven to 450 and prepare pizza stone.

Mix tapioca flour, coconut flour, and salt.

Pour in olive oil and water.

Add in egg and stir well.

Dough should be a little sticky, form into a ball and empty unto a hard surface sprinkled with tapioca flour.

Knead 1-3 minutes or until it forms a non-sticky ball.

Transfer unto parchment parch and with a rolling pin dusted with tapioca powder roll out dough to a 12-14-inch crust. If needed dust rolling pin or pizza with more tapioca flour. However, stay mindful of how much is used as to much will make it dense.

Transfer rolled out dough to prepared pizza stone and bake 12-15 minutes.

Chicken Chow Mein

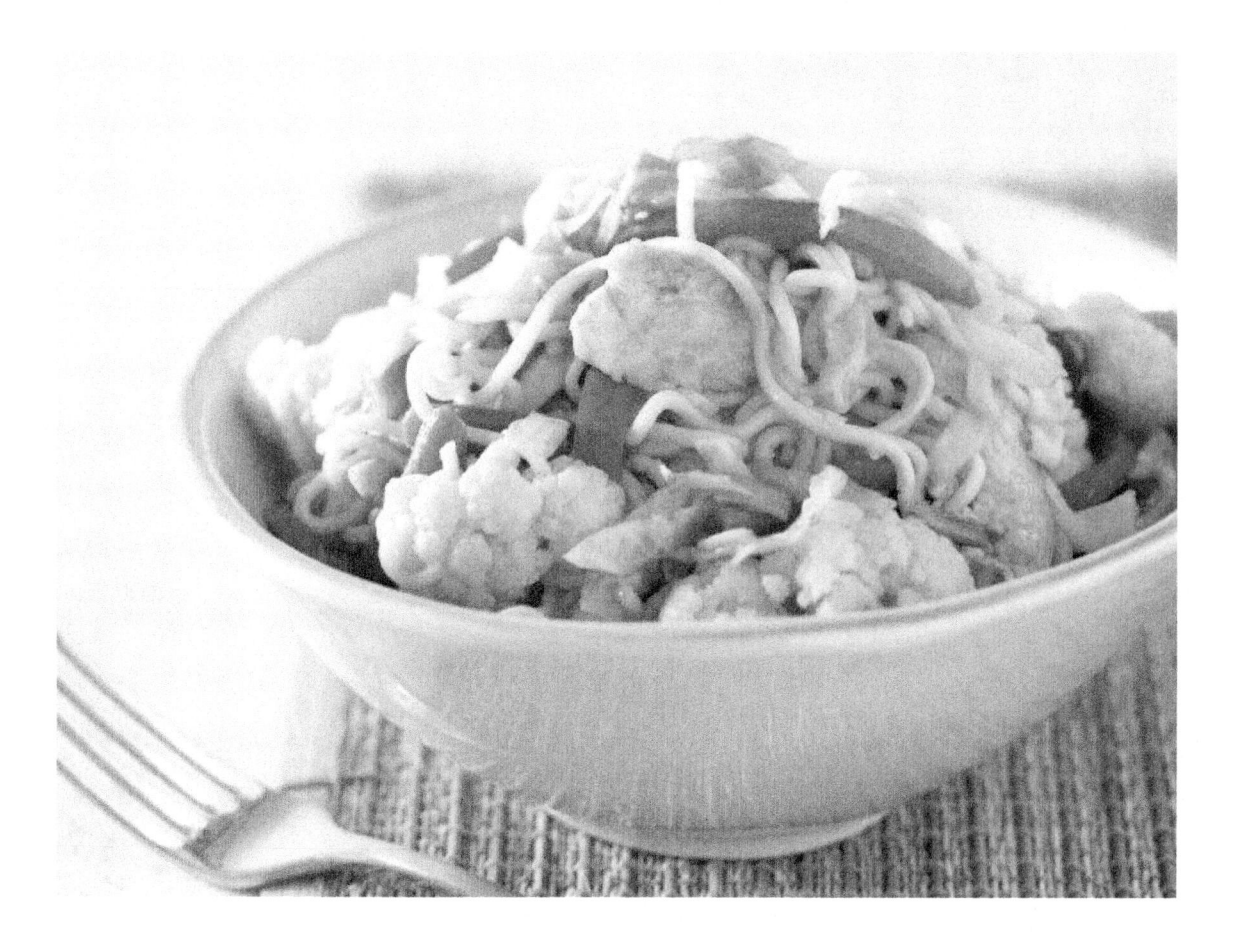

Excellent meat for tacos! Makes approx. 4-6 cups.

Ingredients:

- 3 tsp olive oil or avocado oil
- 1 cup worth sliced chicken strips
- ½ cup cauliflower florets
- 1/3 cup sliced shiitake mushrooms
- 1/2 teaspoon paprika
- 1/2 teaspoon sweet ginger
- 1/4 teaspoon garlic powder
- 1/3 teaspoon onion powder
- 1/3 teaspoon oregano
- ½ cup rice
- 1 can Chow Mein Vegetables

Directions:

Preheat 400 lining it with aluminum foil.

Meanwhile mix smoked paprika, chili powder, garlic powder, onion powder, oregano.

Place cauliflower and sliced mushrooms on sheet drizzle with oil and roast 18-22 minutes or until edges of cauliflower starts to turn at edges.

Sweet Smoky Chicken Kabobs

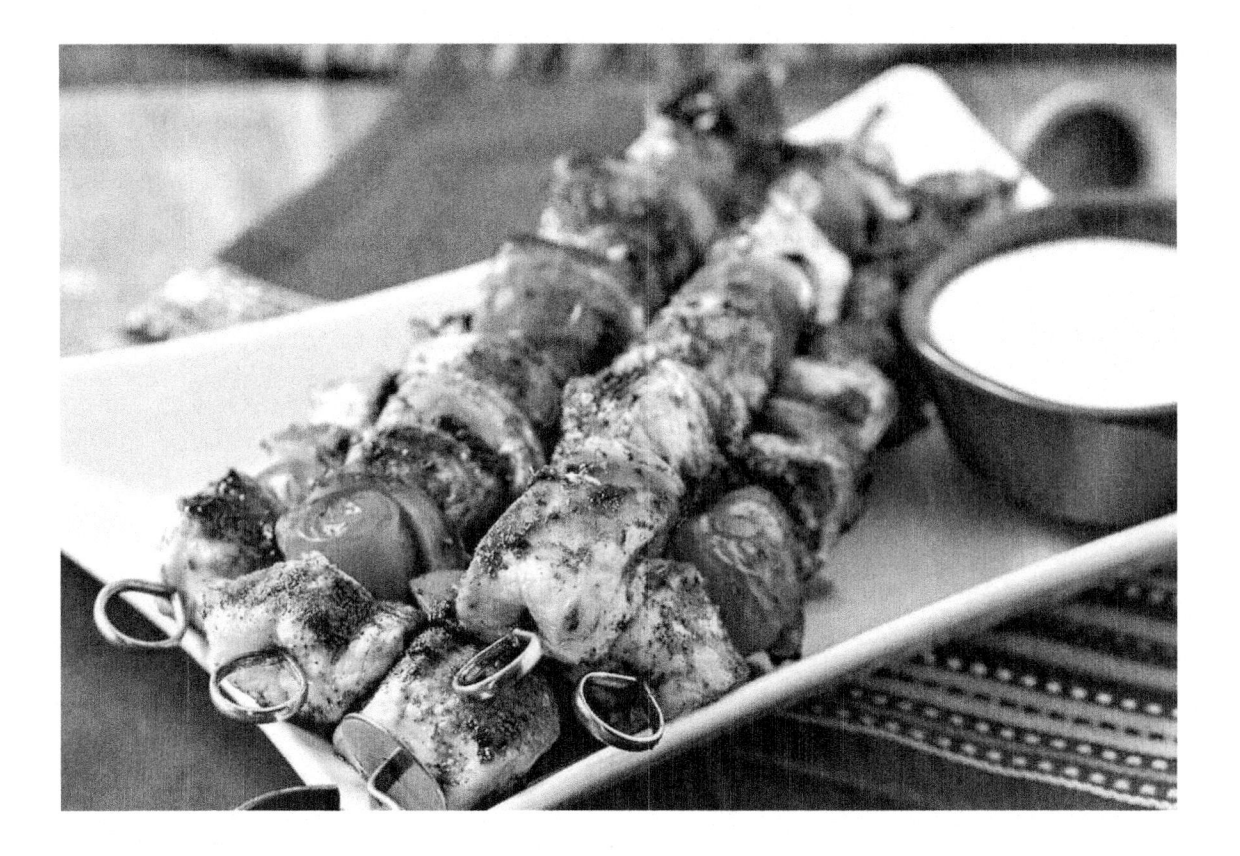

Never eat raw or pink chicken! Makes 2 servings.

Ingredients:

- 1 tablespoon olive oil or coconut oil more for drizzling
- 1/3 cup onion, diced
- 1 clove garlic thinly sliced
- 1/3 cup diced red bell pepper flakes
- ½ tsp liquid smoke
- ½ tsp paprika
- Salt and Pepper for sprinkling
- 1 cup 1x2 chunked chicken
- Olive oil spray
- 4 medium sized skewers soaked in cold water 30 minutes before grilling

Directions:

In marinating dish combine oil, onion, garlic, red bell peppers, smoked paprika, turmeric or cayenne powder, salt, and pepper.

Marinate chicken cubes in refrigerator 30 minutes to 1 hour.

Thread chicken cubes on soaked skewers.

Spray with olive oil.

Broil 4-5 minutes, flip, and repeat.

Burger Bake

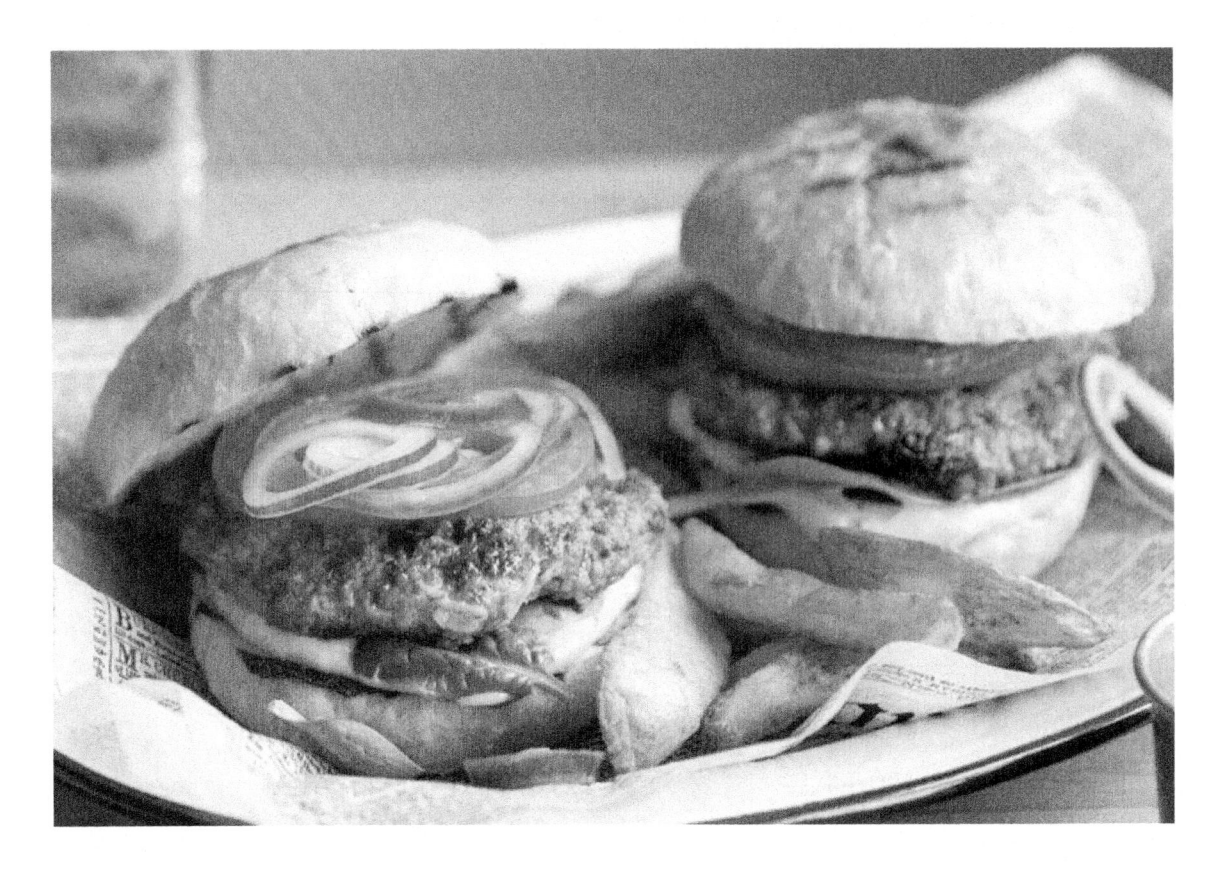

Add in shredded cheddar and make it cheeseburger casserole! Makes 2 servings.

Ingredients:

- 3 scallions, sliced
- ½ cup organic, low sodium black beans
- 1 cup browned and drained ground beef
- 1/3 cup diced mushrooms
- 1/3 tablespoon organic tomato paste
- ½-2/3 cup petite diced no-salt added tomatoes with juice
- 1/2 tbs fresh thyme
- ½ Tbsp chopped cilantro (optional)
- 1 cup water or chicken stock
- ½ cup brown rice
- 1/4 Tbsp basil
- 1/4 Tbsp parsley

Directions:

In pot warmed over medium high heat add sliced scallions, burger, blackbeans, mushrooms, tomato paste, tomatoes, thyme, liquid, rice, basil, parsley.

Bring to a boil, reduce heat, cover, simmer 10-12 minutes.

Artic Ranch Fajita Bowl

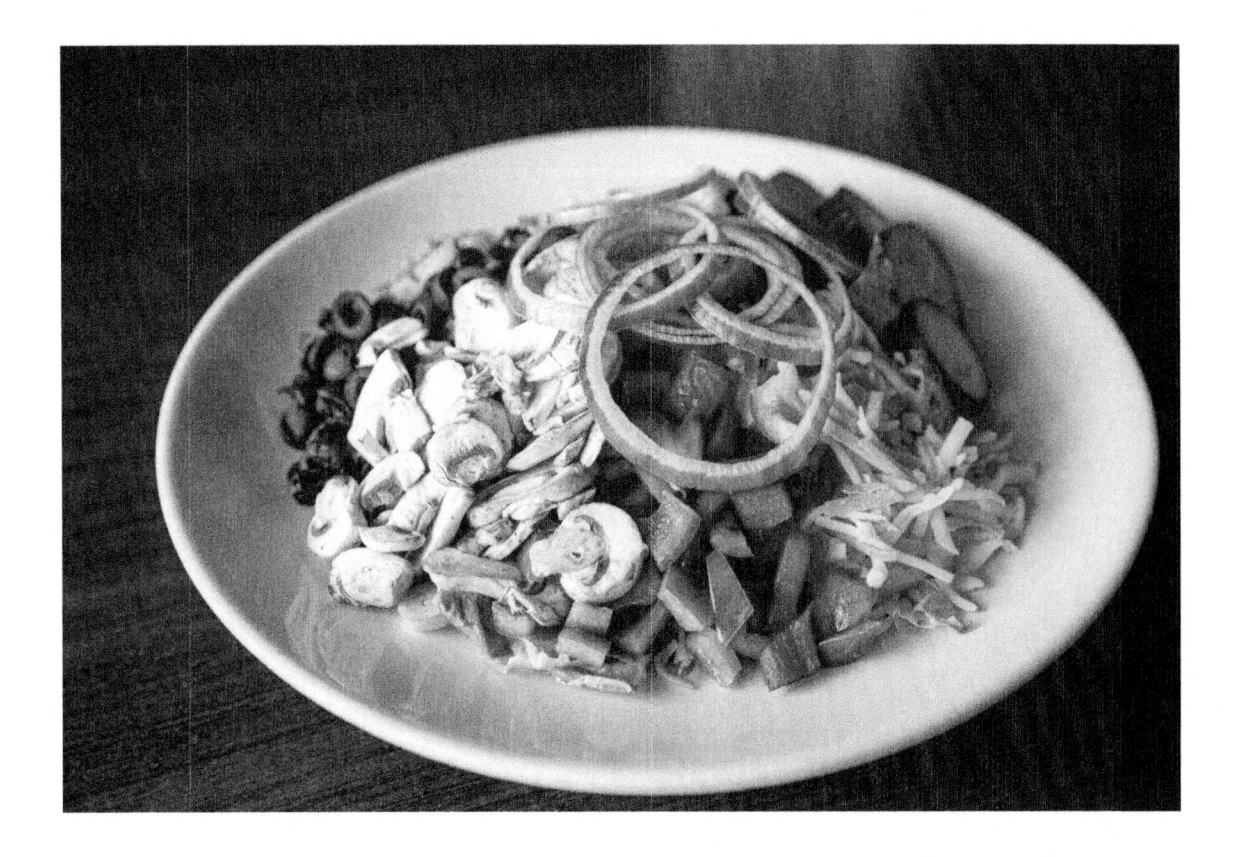

Lots of different chips not labeled as g.f. are ok. Look for corn or potato flour! Makes 2 servings.

Ingredients:

- 3 scallions, sliced
- ½ cup organic, low sodium black beans
- 1 cup browned and drained ground beef
- 1/3 cup diced mushrooms
- 1/3 tablespoon organic tomato paste
- ½-2/3 cup petite diced no-salt added tomatoes with juice
- 1 pack ranch seasoning
- 1 bay leaf
- ½ Tbsp chopped cilantro (optional)
- 1/3 cup water or chicken stock
- Broken tortilla chips (example Doritos)

Directions:

In pot warmed over medium high heat add sliced scallions, burger, blackbeans, mushrooms, tomato paste, tomatoes, ranch seasoning, bay leaf, liquid.

Bring to a boil, reduce heat, cover, simmer 10-12 minutes.

Serve over broken chips.

Cauli-Stuffed Peppers

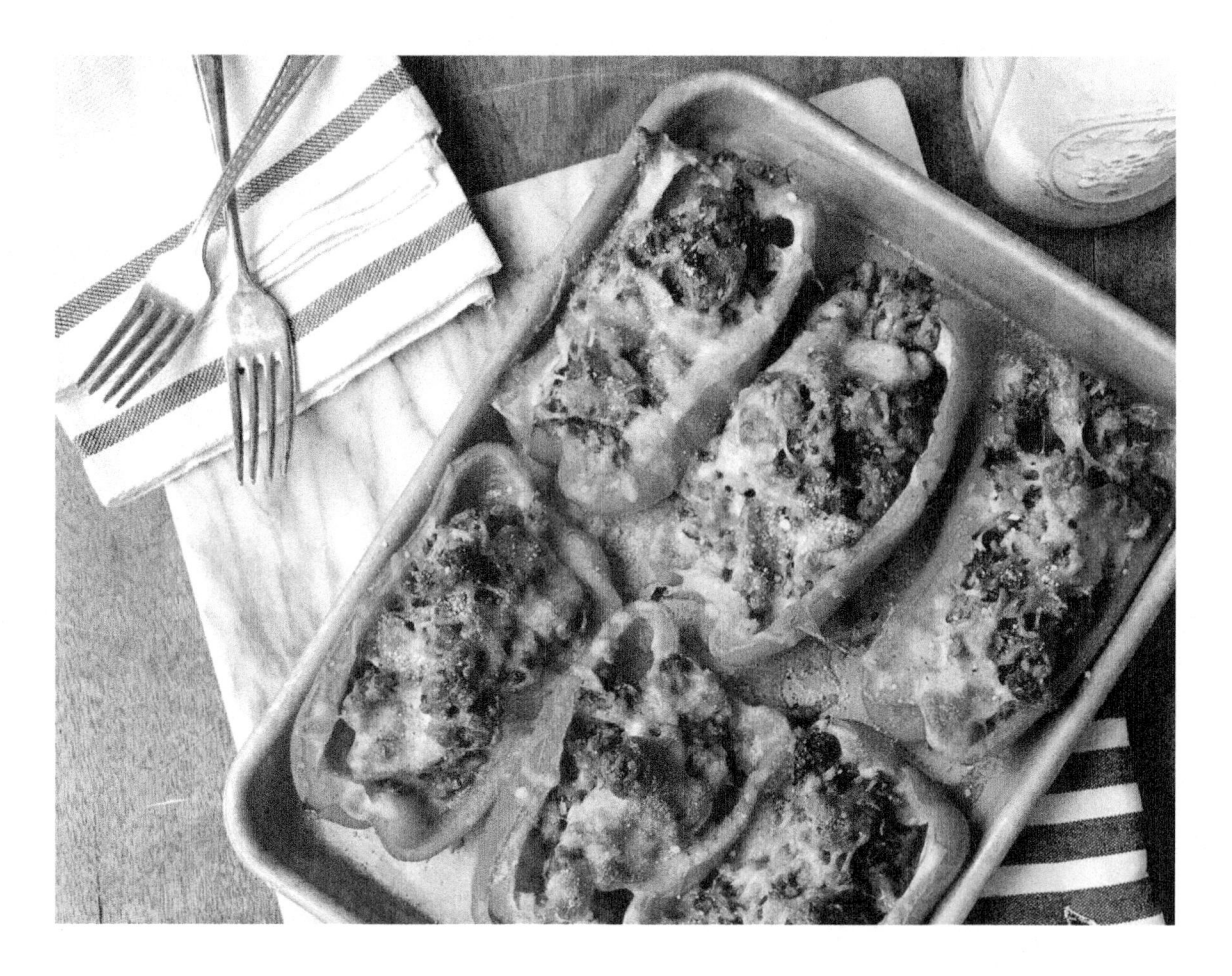

They'll forget it is good for them!! Makes 2 servings,

Ingredients:

- 1 cup cauliflower rice
- ½ cup ground turkey or chicken, browned and drained
- 1/2 teaspoons olive oil
- 1/3 tablespoon butter or ghee
- 1 tablespoon onion, grated
- 1/2 teaspoon garlic, minced
- 1 teaspoon smoked paprika
- 1/3 teaspoon black pepper
- 1 tablespoon pinenuts
- ¼ Tbsp parsley, chopped
- ¼ Tbsp Italian oregano, diced
- 2 bell peppers; washed, stems and seeds removed
- 1-2 cups water

Directions:

In a skillet warmed over medium-high heat add olive oil, butter, onion, garlic, paprika, pepper, cauliflower, protein, pinenuts, parsley, oregano and sauté 1-2 minutes

Spoon cauliflower rice in peppers and place in crockpot.

Pour liquid around peppers.

Cook on high 45 minutes – 1 hour.

G.F. Po Boy

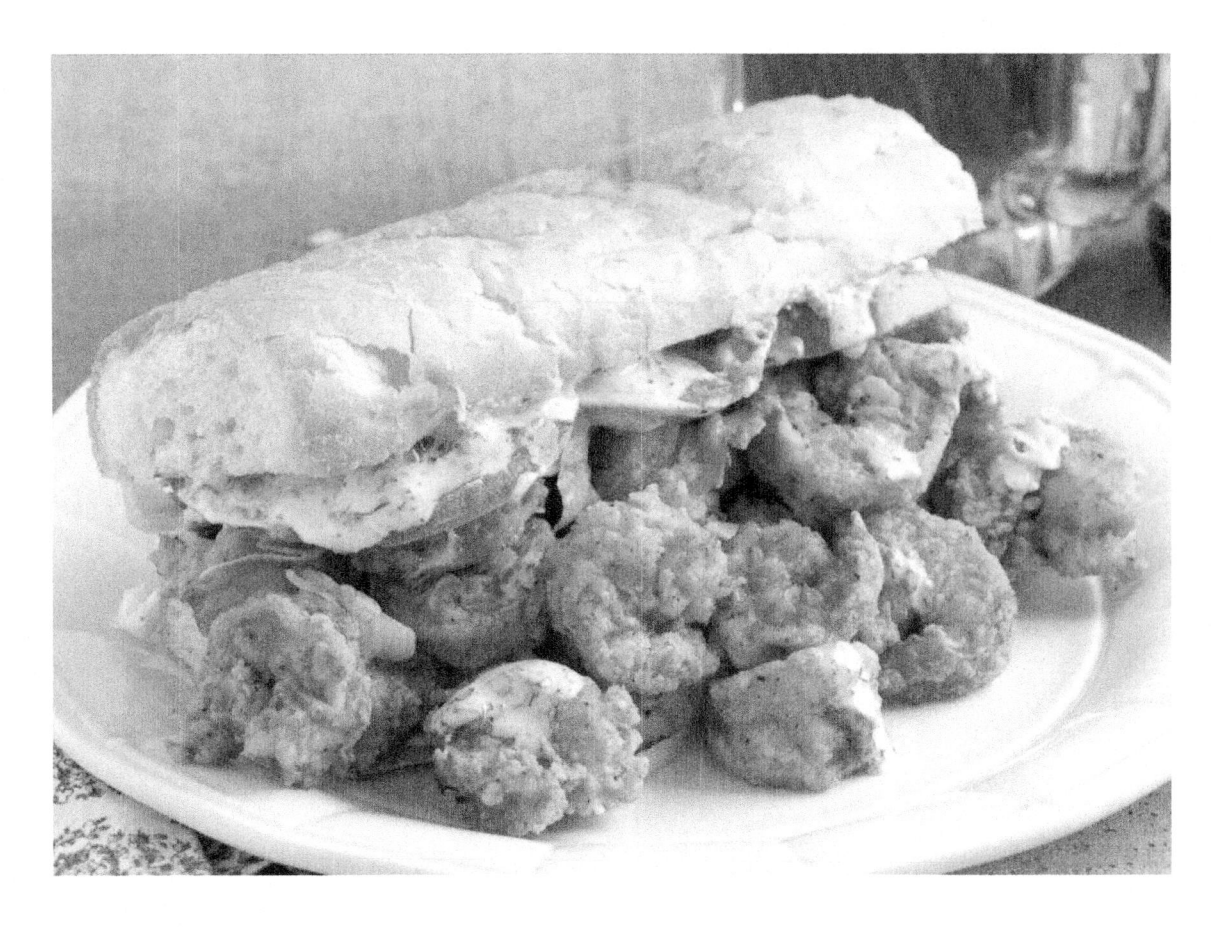

A taste of NOLA! Makes 2 servings.

Ingredients:

- 2 cups shrimp, peeled and deveined
- 1/4 cup + 2 Tbsp mayonnaise
- 4-6 dashes hot sauce
- 1 cup fine yellow corn grits, aka polenta
- 3/4 teaspoon no-salt Cajun seasoning
- 2 g.f. baguettes/hoagie rolls
- Mayonnaise to spread
- ½ cup shredded lettuce
- Sliced pickles or banana peppers
- 1 tomato, sliced

Directions:

Preheat oven to 400 and prepare baking sheet.

Mix together mayo and hot sauce.

In a separate bowl, combine grits and Cajun seasoning.

Dip shrimp in mayo mix then dunk into grit mix. Making sure shrimp is thoroughly coated.

Place shrimp on baking sheet and mist with olive oil.

Cook 12-15 minutes.

If using a baguette, toast as directed.

Crispy, Baked Gluten Free Fish Sticks

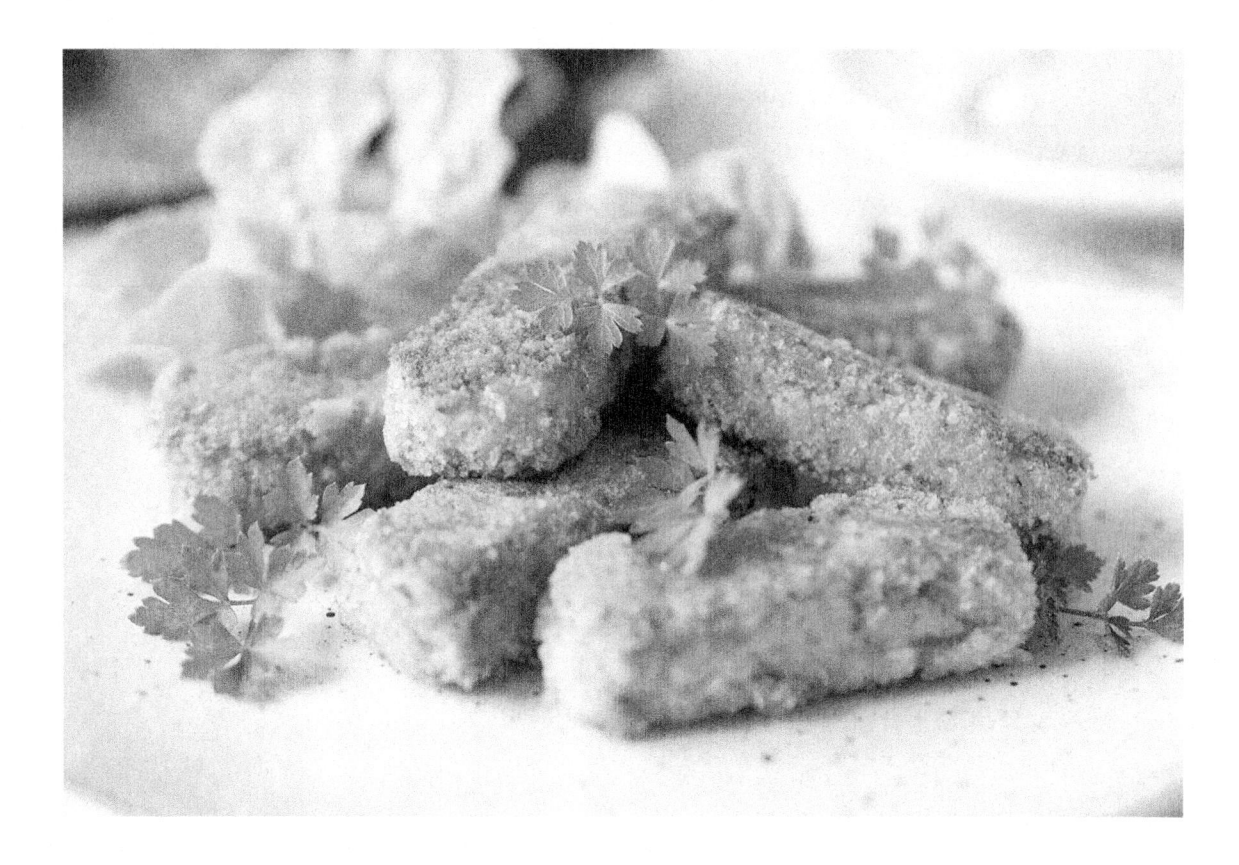

Mix in your favorite spices! Makes 8-10 fish sticks

Ingredients:

- 1 filet of cod, sliced
- 2 eggs, beaten
- 1 ½ cup g.f. 1-1 all-purpose flour
- 1 ½ cup g.f. plain breadcrumbs

Directions:

Preheat oven to 400 and prepare baking tray.

Dip fish sticks into beaten egg and knock off excess.

Dip fish sticks into flour and shake off excess.

Dip fish sticks into g.f. breadcrumbs and shake off excess.

Bake 20-25 minutes.

Quick Protein Noodles

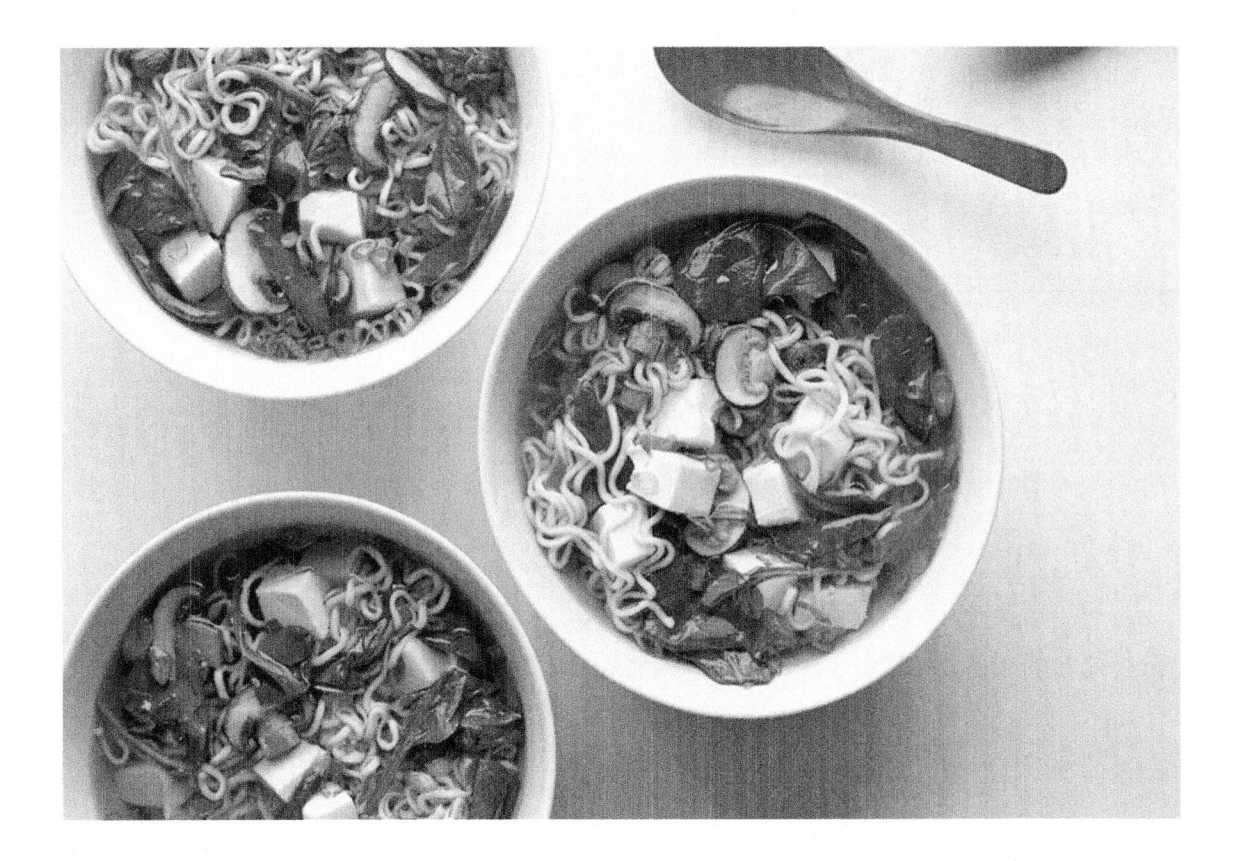

Great for that extra boost! Makes 2 servings.

Ingredients:

- 1/2 teaspoon sesame oil
- ½ tablespoon olive oil
- 1/4 cup finely chopped spinach, washed
- ½ teaspoon garlic, minced
- ½ tsp red pepper flakes (optional)
- ½ cup low sodium garbanzo or blackbeans
- 1/2 cup edamame or green/yellow beans
- 1/3 cup chicken or veggie stock (water works too)
- 1/2 cup worth rice noodles, uncooked
- ½ package tofu or a protein (optional)
- 2 Tbsp chopped fresh herbs

Directions:

In Dutch oven add sesame oil, olive oil, spinach, minced garlic, red pepper flakes, beans, stock and sauté 1 minute.

Add in cubed tofu, edamame, stock or water, uncooked rice noodles. Stir well.

Bring to a boil, cover, reduce heat, let simmer 20-25

Easy G.F. Eggroll Wrappers

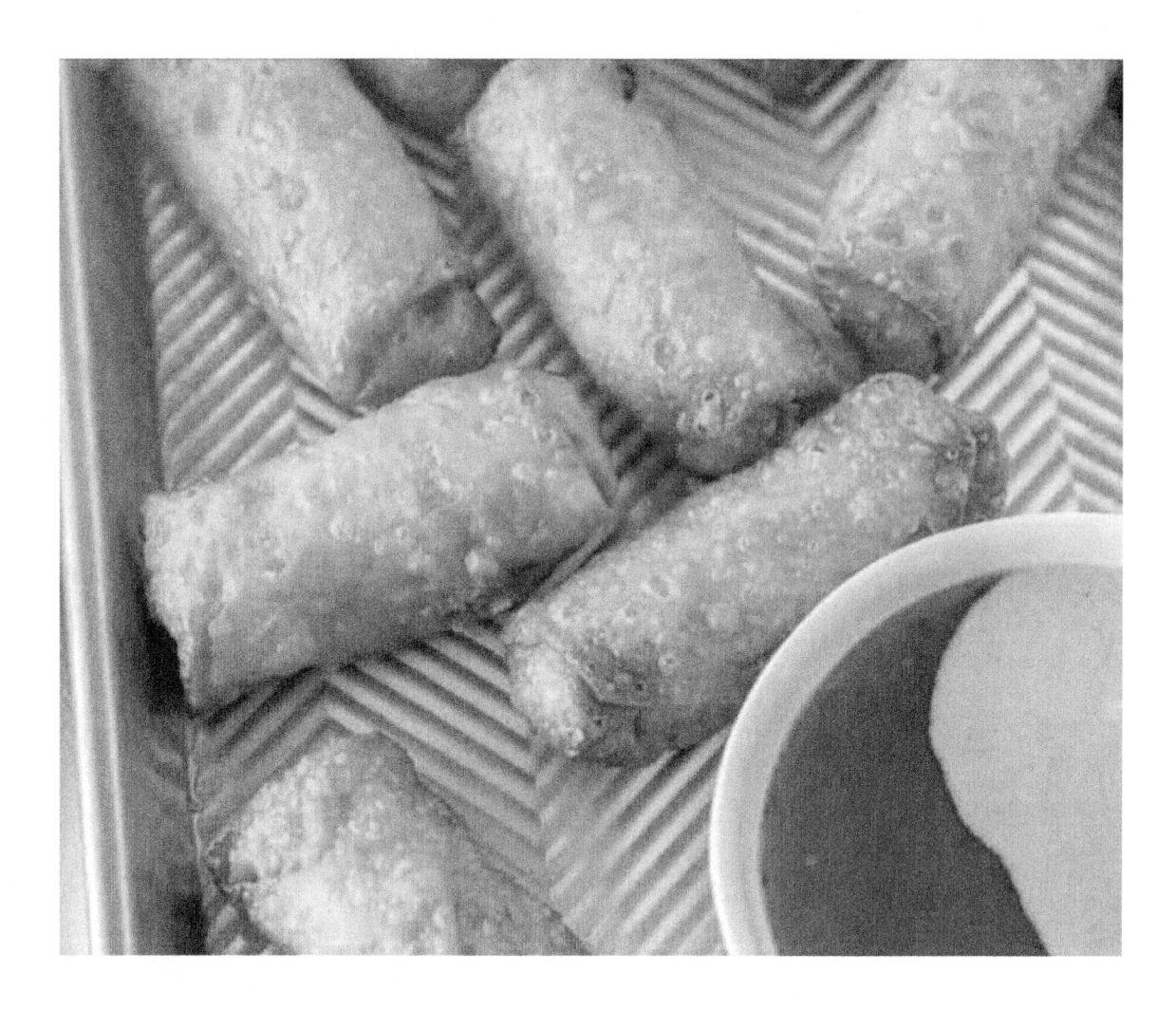

Oh, so worth it! Makes

Ingredients:

- 1 1/3 cups cornstarch (coconut flour, potato starch, tapioca flour or anything similar works)
- 1 1/3 cups brown rice flour (can sub with g.f. white or oat flour)
- 1/3 teaspoon xanthan gum (if not already in the flour)
- 1/4 teaspoon salt
- 2 eggs
- 3/4 cup water

Directions:

Combine starch, flour, gum, salt.

Whisk together eggs and water then pour into starch mix.

Stir until dough forms a ball.

Sprinkle counter/work surface with starch and roll 1/3 dough to preferred thickness (we opted for approx. ¼-inch thick.

Cut into 6x6 sections and place on prepared baking sheet.

If not using immediately, cover with damp towel and store in a cool, dark place.

When ready to cook, fill and roll, then fry to a golden brown 2-3 minutes per side.

Cabbage Eggrolls

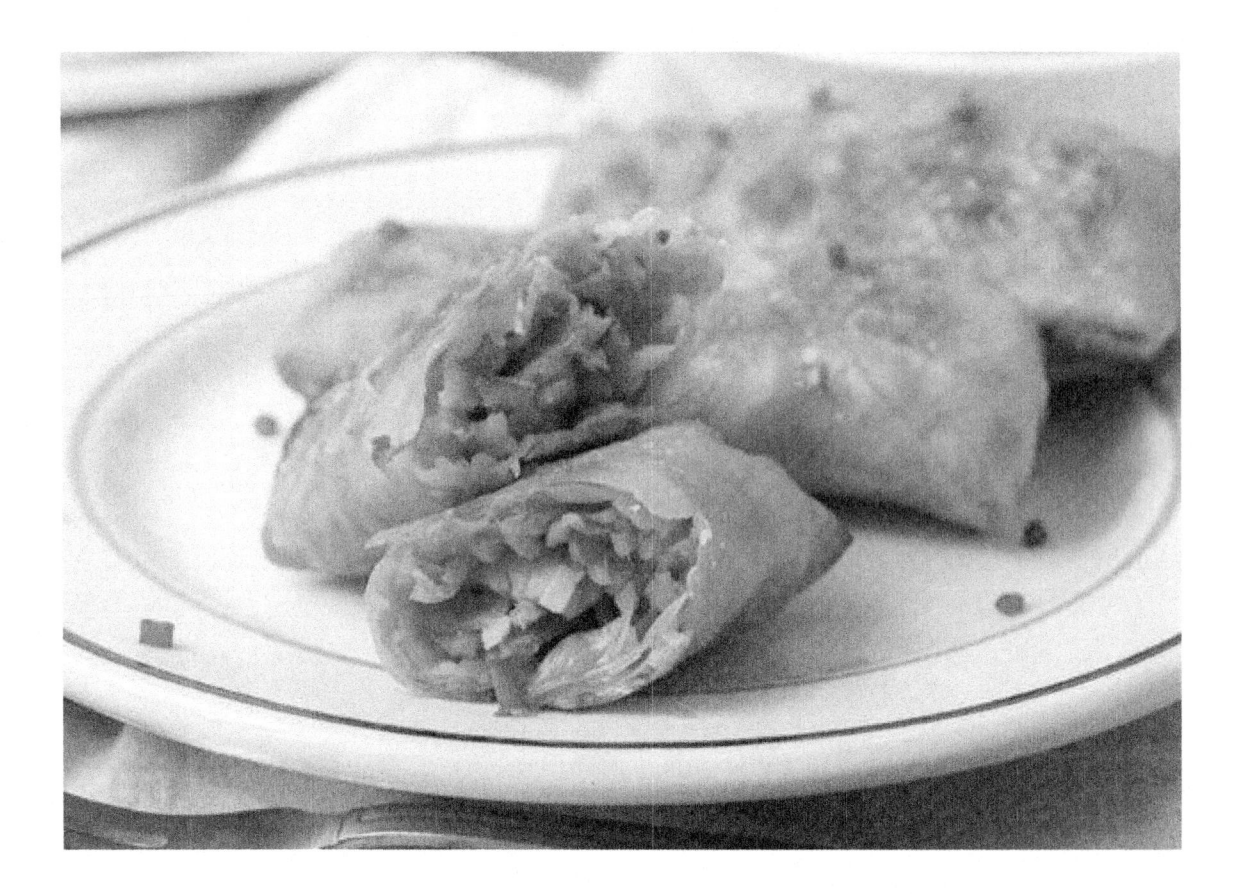

Serve with gluten free biscuits or spring rolls! Makes 18-24 servings.

Ingredients:

- ¼ teaspoon rice vinegar
- 1/4 cup olive oil
- 1-2 drops chili oil or paste
- ½ Tbsp thyme
- 1 diced scallion
- 1 tsp minced garlic
- 1 tsp minced or grated onion
- ½ Tbsp shredded carrots
- 2/3 cup shredded cabbage

Directions:

In skillet mix olive oil, wine vinegar, chili oil, thyme, diced scallions, garlic, onion.

Sauté 30-45 seconds, swirling oils around surface area.

Stir in cabbage and carrots.

Spoon into Easy G.F. Wrapper

Cauliflower Gnocchi

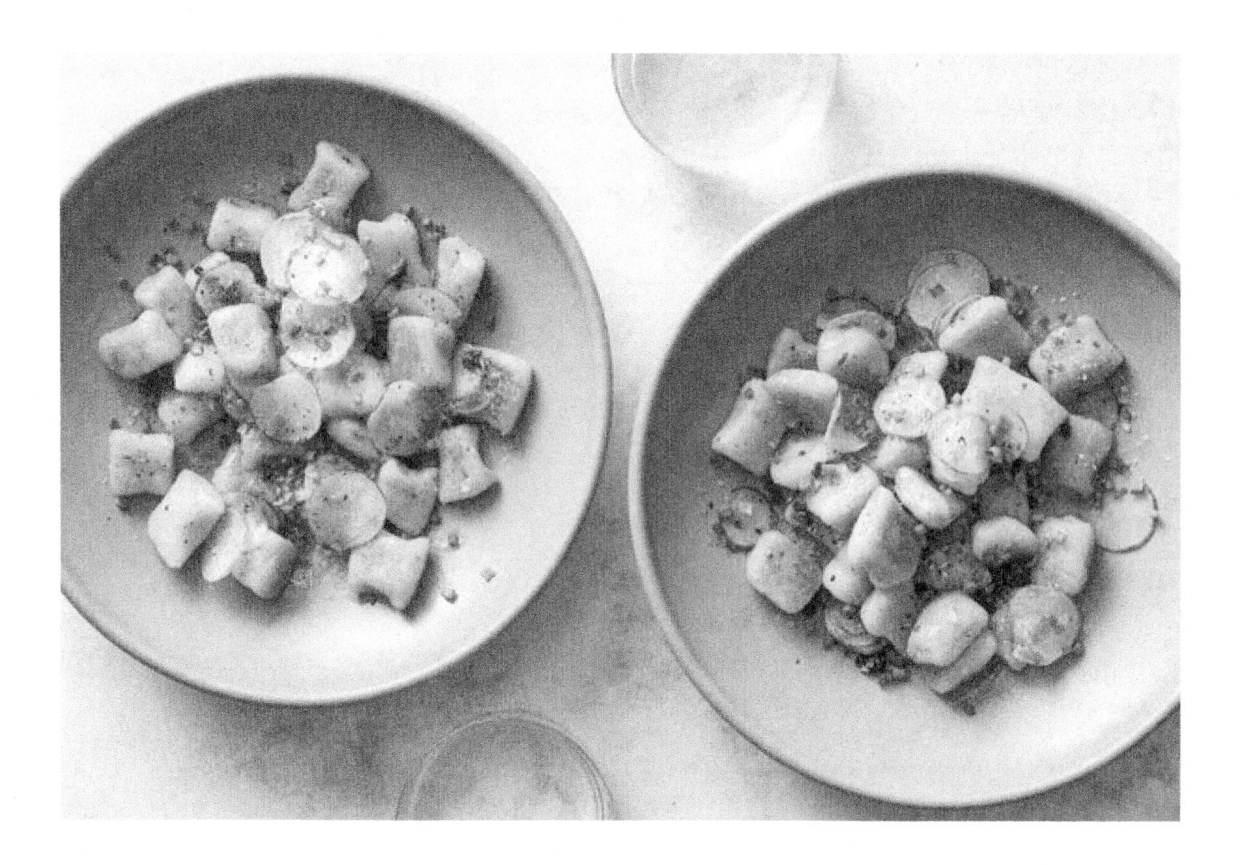

Gnocchi is a great for sneaking veggie's into kids' diet! Makes 2 servings.

Ingredients:

- 1 cup cauliflower, florets
- 1/2 Tbsp cassava flour
- 2 tsp tapioca flour
- ½ teaspoon thyme
- 1 teaspoon garlic, minced
- ½ teaspoon lemon peel

Directions:

Steam cauliflower 5-7 minutes, ring out water, put in blender along with cassava flour and smoked paprika. Blend until mix is smooth.

Roll dough into 1-inch thick tube then cut into four segments, place three in the refrigerator.

Cut each segment into 1-inch pieces, drop them into boiling water and let rise to surface.

Once they have risen, transfer them to baking tray 20 minutes, turn over, cook another 30 minutes.

In skillet over medium-high heat whisk together coconut milk, minced garlic, lemon peel, pepper, tapioca flour. Stirring continuously until smooth and thickens.

Italiano Chicken with Faux Fried Onion Rings

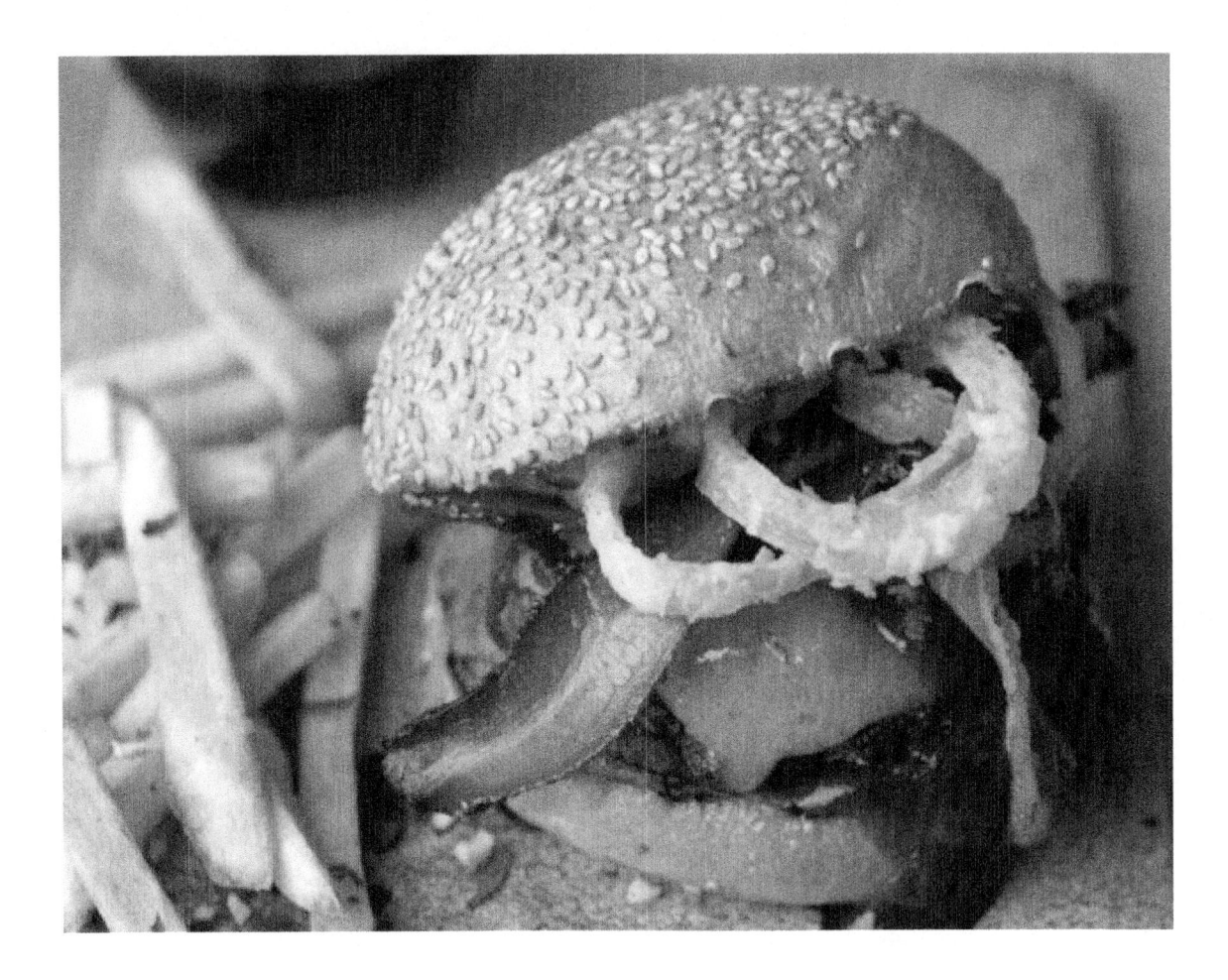

Great on a bun! Makes 2 servings

Ingredients:

- 2 boneless, skinless chicken breasts
- 1 cup g.f.a.p. flour
- 1 cup g.f. breadcrumbs
- 1 tsp Italian seasoning
- ½ tsp garlic powder
- 1/3 tsp smoked paprika
- Olive oil spray
- G.F. hamburger buns
- 1 large onion sliced into rings.

Directions:

Preheat oven to 425 and prepare small baking sheet.

Stir Italian seasoning, garlic powder, and smoked paprika into flour.

Coat breasts and onion rings with flour, shake off excess.

Lay onion rings on plate, cover, store in refrigerator.

Coat breasts with breadcrumbs, shake off excess.

Place both breasts in bottom of pan, cover with aluminum foil, and cook 45 minutes.

Remove foil, top with onion rings and spray again.

Cook another 15-30 minutes depending on breast size (extended cooking times may have to adjust onion cooking times too)

Sweet Heat Fish Sticks

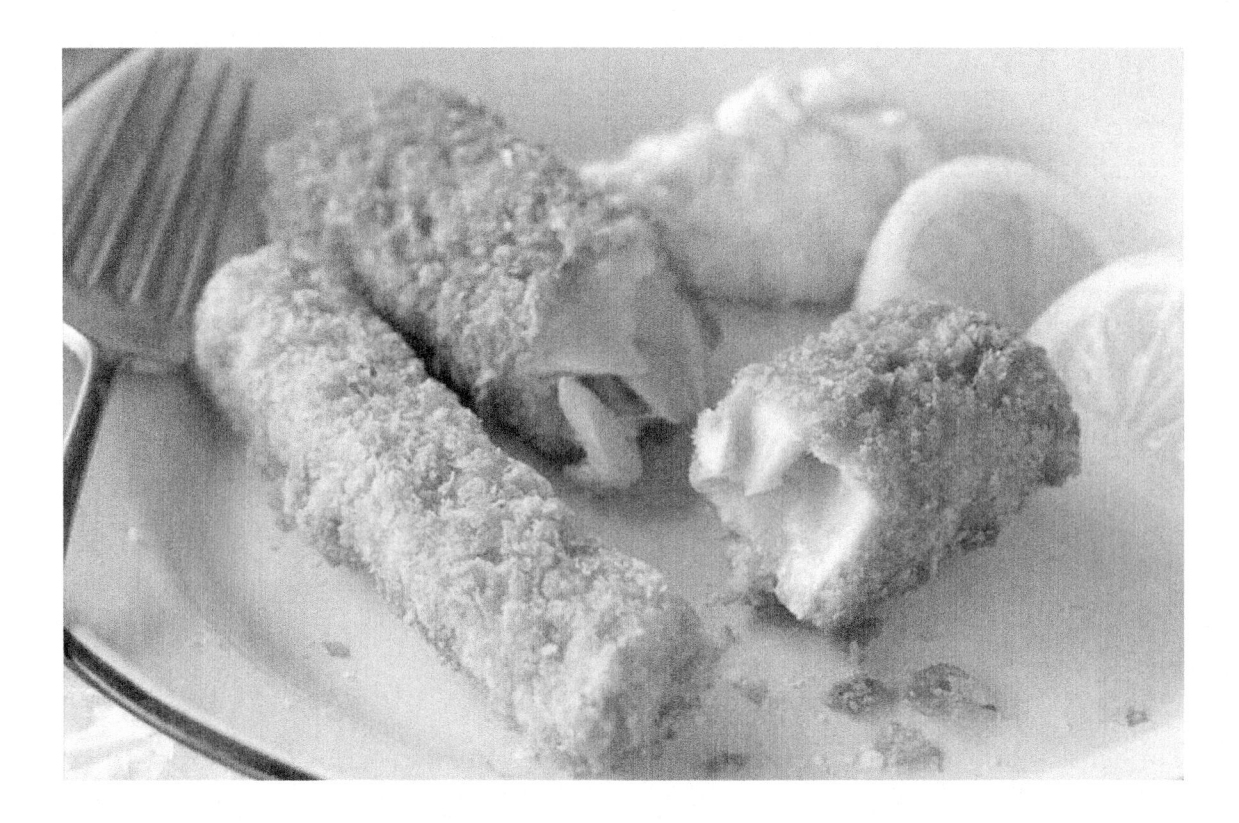

Great on shrimp too! Makes 2 servings

Ingredients:

- 12 strips of cod or fish sticks
- ½ cup g.f. breadcrumbs
- ½ cup g.f.a.p. flour
- ½ tsp sweet paprika
- ½ tsp red pepper flakes

Directions:

Preheat oven to 400 and line baking sheet with aluminum foil.

Set up breading station.

Mix into flour sweet paprika and red pepper flakes.

Coat fish in flour, shake off excess.

Coat fish in breadcrumbs, shake off excess.

Layout sticks, mist with olive oil, and bake 20-30 minutes

Spirals in a Dairy-Free Sauce

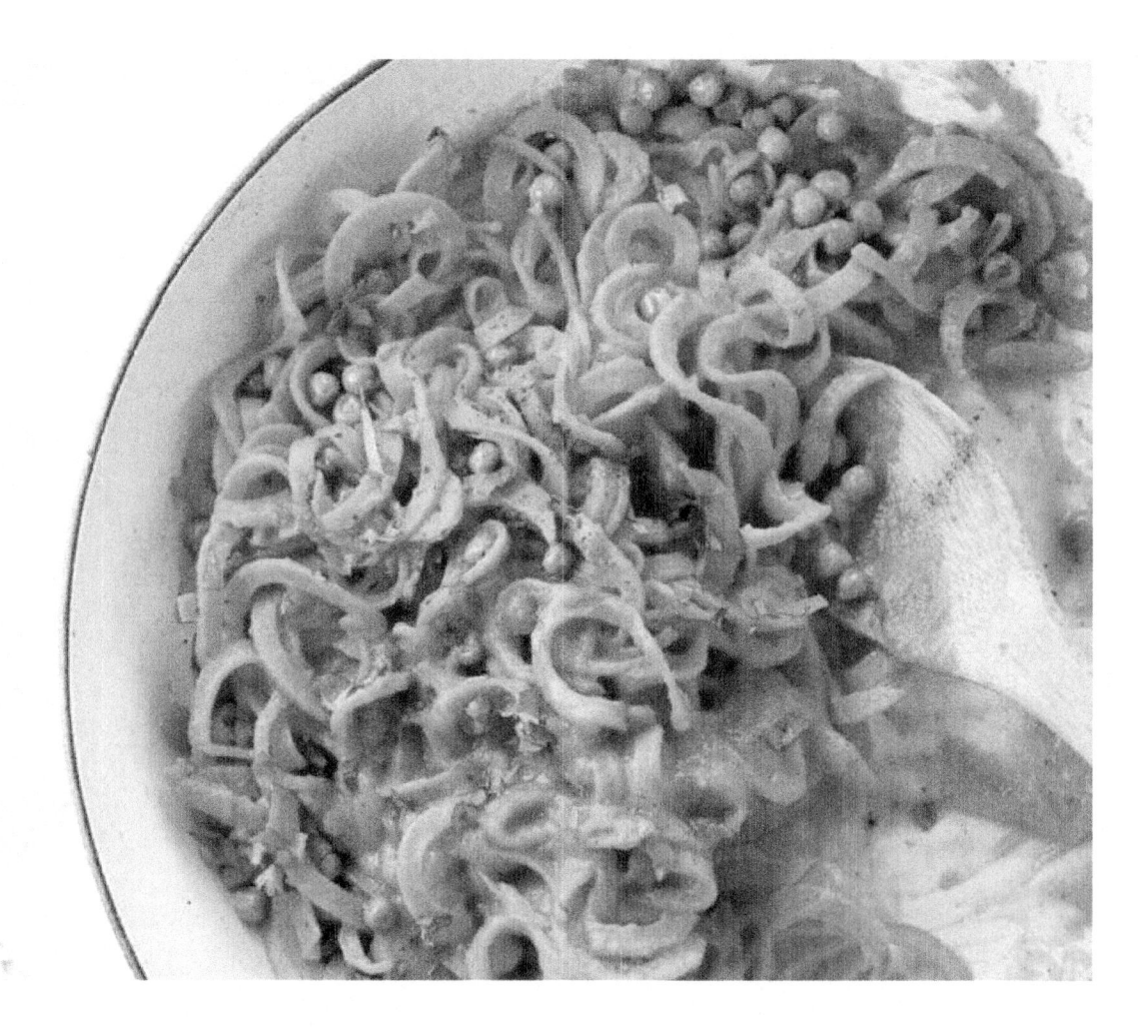

Throw some bell peppers or jalapenos in! Makes 2 servings.

Ingredients:

- 1 cup sweet potato spirals
- 1/2 tablespoon butter or ghee
- 1/3 Tbsp onion, grated
- 1/2 teaspoon garlic, minced
- 1/4 cup coconut milk
- 1 1/2 teaspoons tapioca flour
- 1/4 teaspoons thyme, diced
- 1/3 teaspoon rosemary
- 1/4 teaspoon red pepper flakes

Directions:

Mix sweet potato spirals, oil and flour together.

In skillet butter melt the add julienned onions. Turn heat to medium-low and let onions sweat 10 minutes.

Whisk in garlic and coconut milk, stirring constantly for 30 seconds. Whisk in tapioca flour, diced rosemary, diced oregano, red pepper flakes. Bring to a low boil for 1-2 minutes constantly stirring.

Pour over spirals.

Baked Chicken Tenders

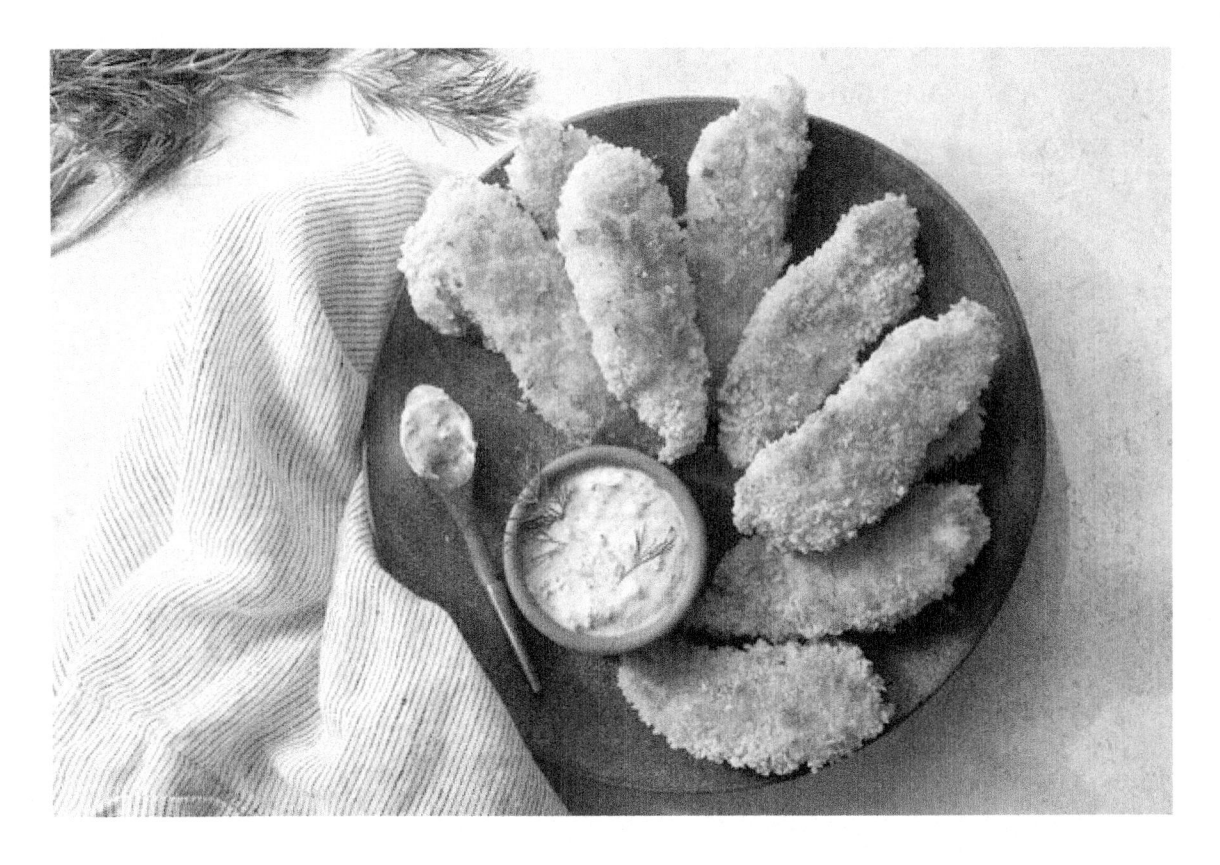

Make a great dipping sauce to accommodate these delicious tenders! Makes 2 serving.

Ingredients:

- 1 cup g.f.a.p. flour
- 1/4 teaspoon lemon peel
- 1/3 tsp red pepper flakes
- 1/3 tsp sweet ginger
- 1/2 cup toasted coconut flakes
- 4 chicken tenders
- 1 cup gluten free breadcrumbs
- Olive oil for drizzling

Directions:

Preheat oven to 400 and prepare 9x11 dish.

Mix into flour lemon peel, sweet ginger, and red pepper flakes

Dredge chicken through breadcrumbs, lay on tray and drizzle with olive oil.

Bake 15 minutes, flip and repeat.

G.F. Mediterranean Quinoa Salad

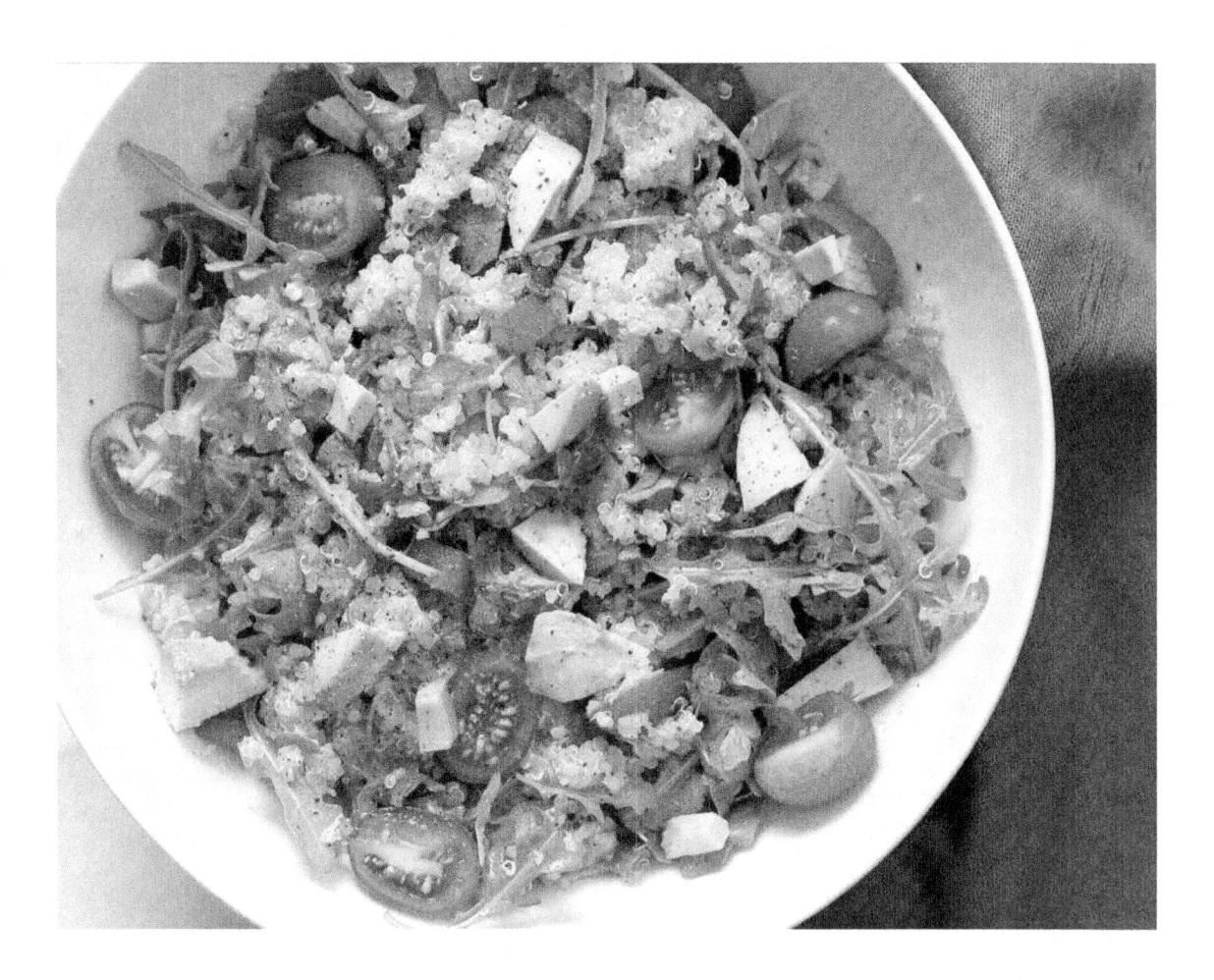

Try various stocks! Makes 2 servings.

Ingredients:

- 1 Tbsp butter
- ¼ cup julienned onions (optional)
- 1/3 cup quinoa
- 1/3 can organic whole kernel corn drained
- ½ cup avocado
- Juice of ½ lemon
- 1 tsp Italian or Greek seasoning

Directions:

In Dutch oven combine olive oil and onions over medium to medium-low heat and sauté 3-4 minutes.

Stir in quinoa, corn, avocado, lemon juice, seasoning.

Bring to a boil, reduce temp, cover, simmer 10-12 minutes.

Broiled Shrimp

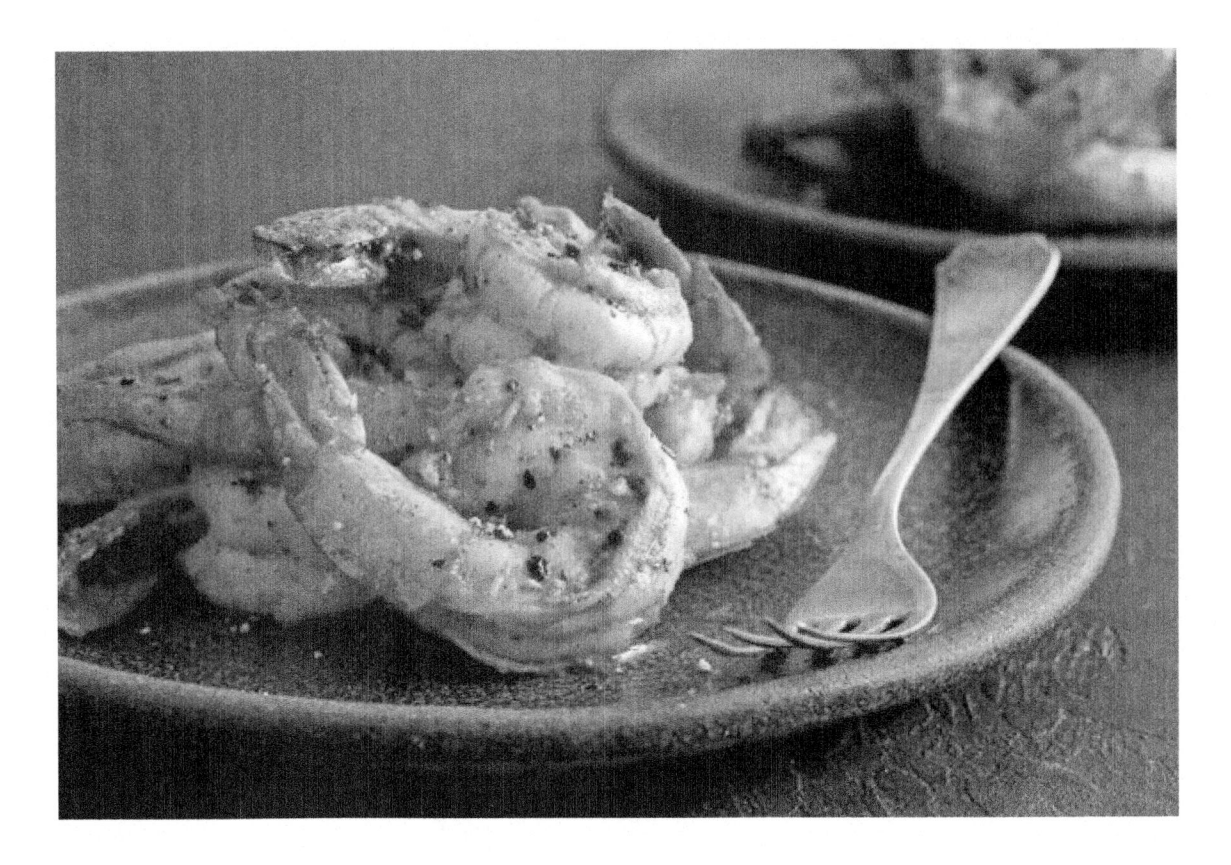

Scallops work too! Makes 20 shrimp

Ingredients:

- 20 medium or large shrimp
- Salt and pepper
- 1 stick butter melted
- ½ tsp paprika
- 1/3 tsp chicken bouillon granules
- ¼ tsp lemon peel
- ¼ tsp pepper

Directions:

Turn broiler on high and prepare baking sheet.

Melt butter.

Mix paprika, chicken granules, lemon peel, pepper into butter.

Lay shrimp on baking sheet and brush liberally with butter.

Place under broiler 4-5 minutes per-side.

G.F. Baked Chicken Nuggets Cauli-Chips

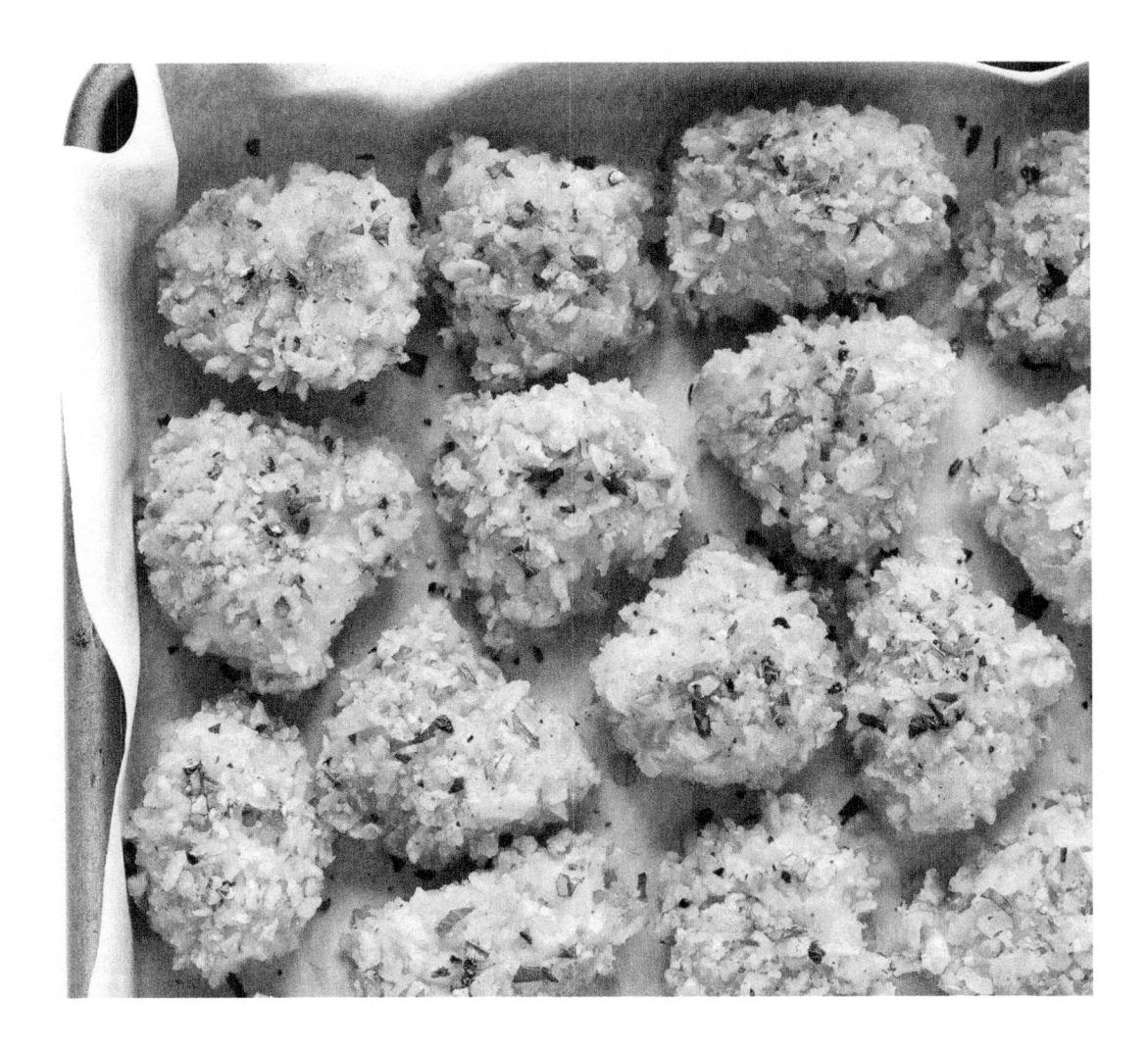

Get creative! How many healthy chips can you think of? Makes 2 servings.

Ingredients:

- 1 large chicken breast
- Olive oil spray
- 2/3 cup gluten free breadcrumbs
- 1 ½ tsp paprika
- 1 cup cauliflower rice
- 2 tablespoon extra-virgin olive oil
- ½ teaspoon garlic powder
- 1 ½ teaspoon Italian seasoning

Directions:

Preheat oven to 350 and prepare muffin tin and lined baking sheet with aluminum foil.

Chop chicken into 1x1 cubes or 'nuggets.'

Mix paprika into g.f. breadcrumbs.

Dredge nuggets through crumbs and lay on baking tray.

Mist with spray bake 15 minutes, flip and repeat.

(due to discrepancies in ovens you might need to try slightly higher and lower temps)

Mix cauliflower rice, e.v. olive oil, minced garlic, diced onion, paprika (optional).

Press into muffin tins and bake 30 minutes.

Store in airtight container in refrigerator and will keep 3-5 days.

Chickpea Chicken Tenders Broccoli Tots

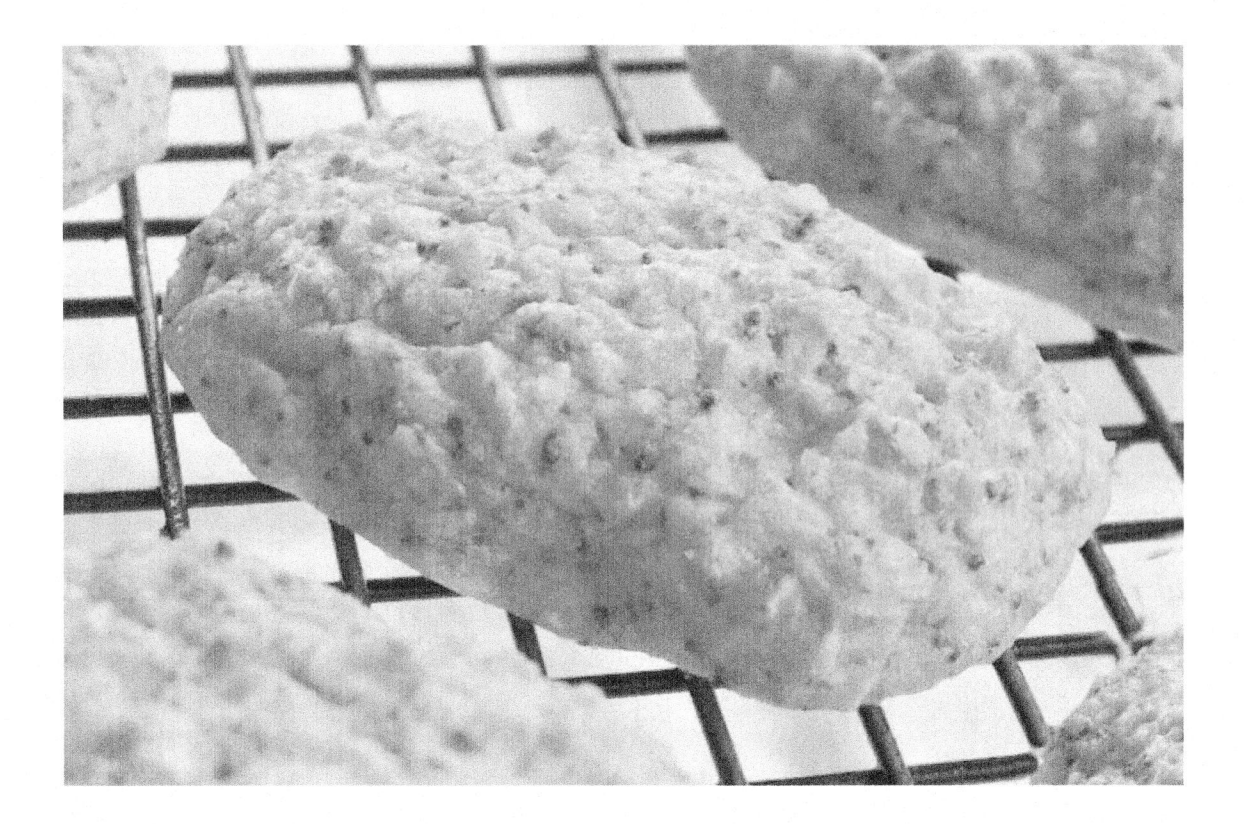

Tots are also good baked! Makes 2 servings.

Ingredients:

- 4-6 chicken tenders
- 1 cup chickpea flour
- Olive oil spray
- 2 cups broccoli mash
- 1/3 cup shredded cheddar cheese
- ½ tsp red pepper flakes (optional)
- 1 tablespoon paprika
- ½ tablespoon garlic powder and parsley

Directions:

Preheat oven to 425, prepare medium sized baking dish and line a baking sheet with aluminum foil.

Coat chicken tenders with chickpea flour, mist with olive oil, bake 35-40 minutes.

Blend together broccoli, cheese, red pepper flakes, paprika, garlic powder and parsley.

Using hands form into tater tots and shallow fry in coconut oil 1-2 minutes per side.

Apple-Cinnamon Pork Chops

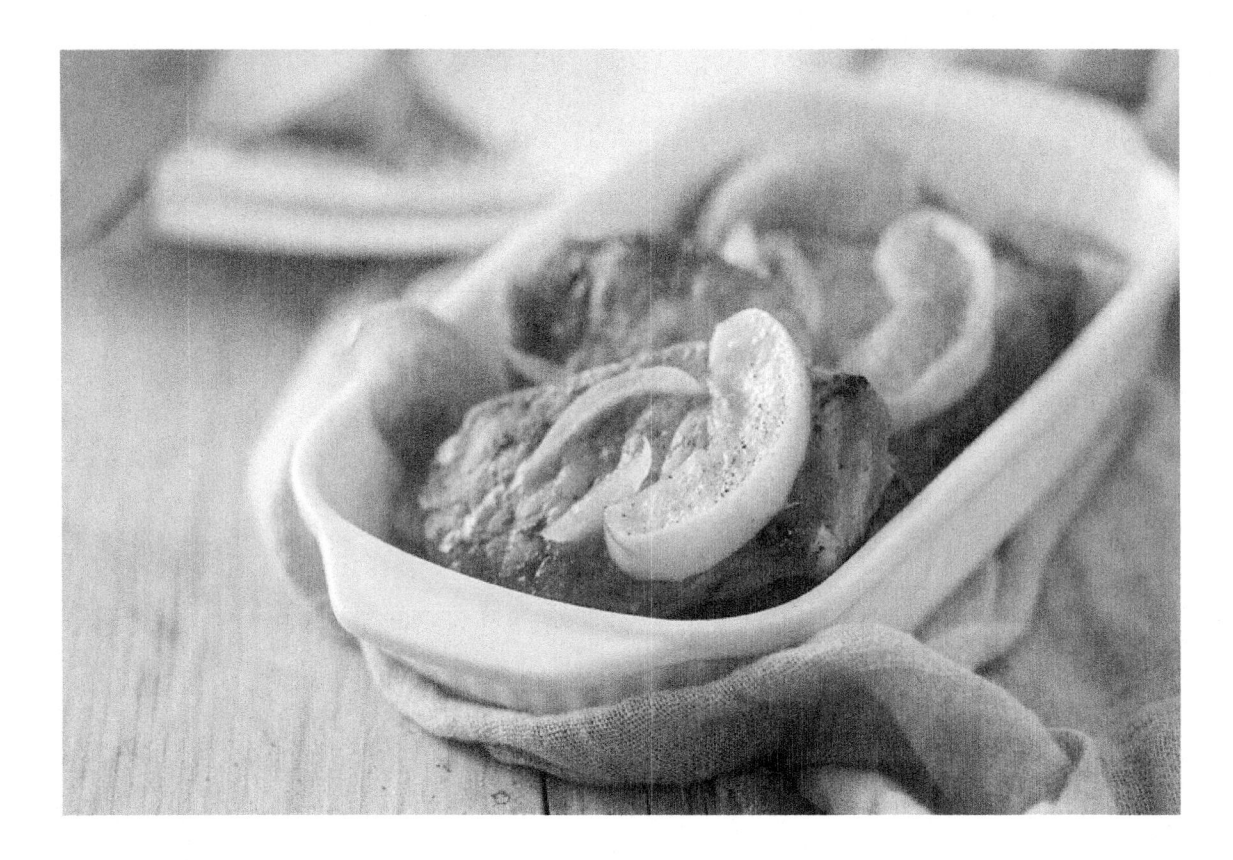

Add a dash of nutmeg and lots of love! Makes 2 servings.

Ingredients:

- ¼ cup melted coconut oil (use more if needed)
- 2 bone-in pork chops
- 1/3 tsp apple pie seasoning
- ½ tsp cinnamon
- ¼ tsp lemon peel
- 1/6 tsp pepper

Directions:

In crockpot add coconut oil, bone-in porkchops, and sprinkle on the apple pie filling and cinnamon. Cook 45 minutes to 1 hour on high.

Transfer to paper towel lined plates.

Before plating dust both sides of pork chops with cinnamon.

Sweet Tots

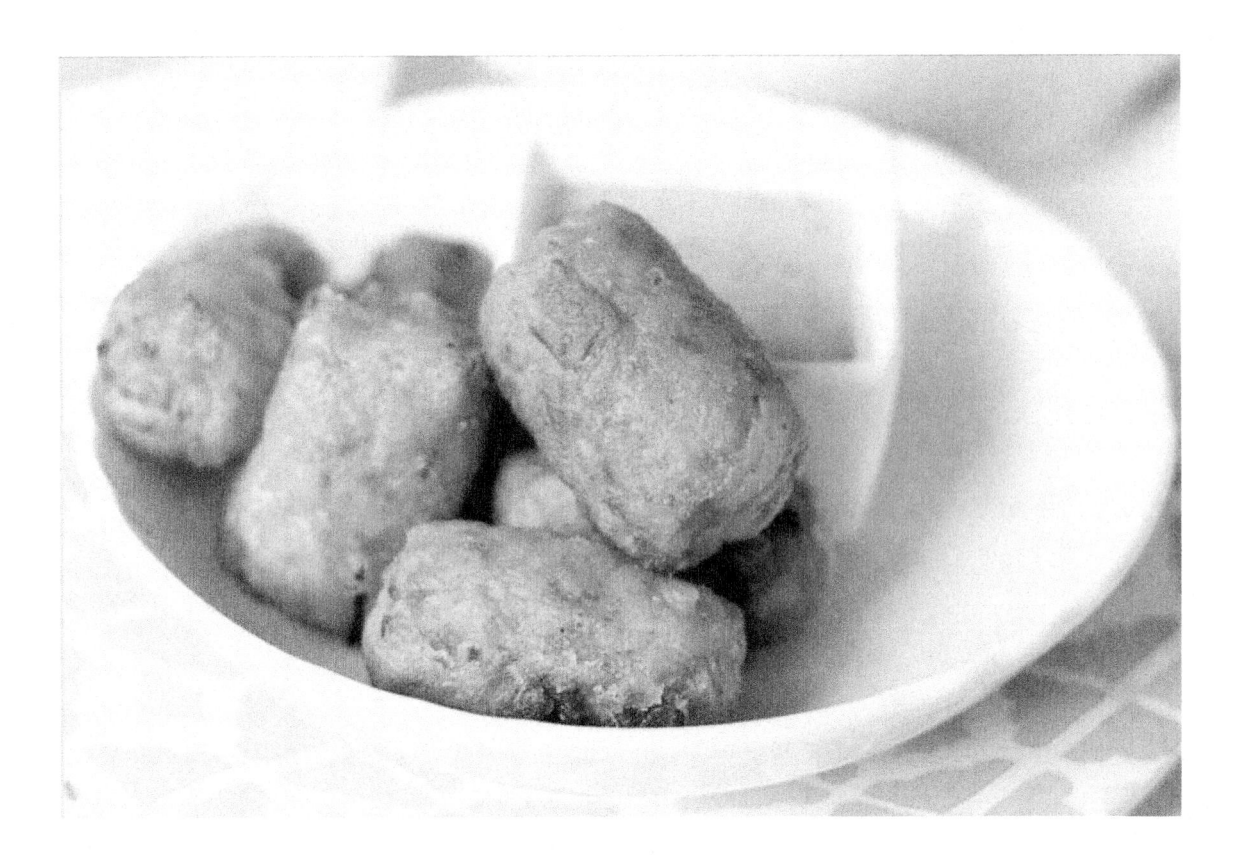

Pumpkin mash works too! Makes 2-4 servings.

Ingredients:

- 1 cup sweet potato mash
- 1/3 tablespoon chili powder
- 1/2 tablespoon paprika
- 1/4 tablespoon cayenne pepper
- 1/3 teaspoon garlic powder and parsley

Directions:

Mix sweet potato, chili powder, paprika, cayenne powder, garlic powder parsley.

With hands form into tater tots.

Lay out on plate.

Sprinkle both sides with spice mixture.

Shallow fry in oil 1-2 minutes per side.

Air Fryer Sweet Tots

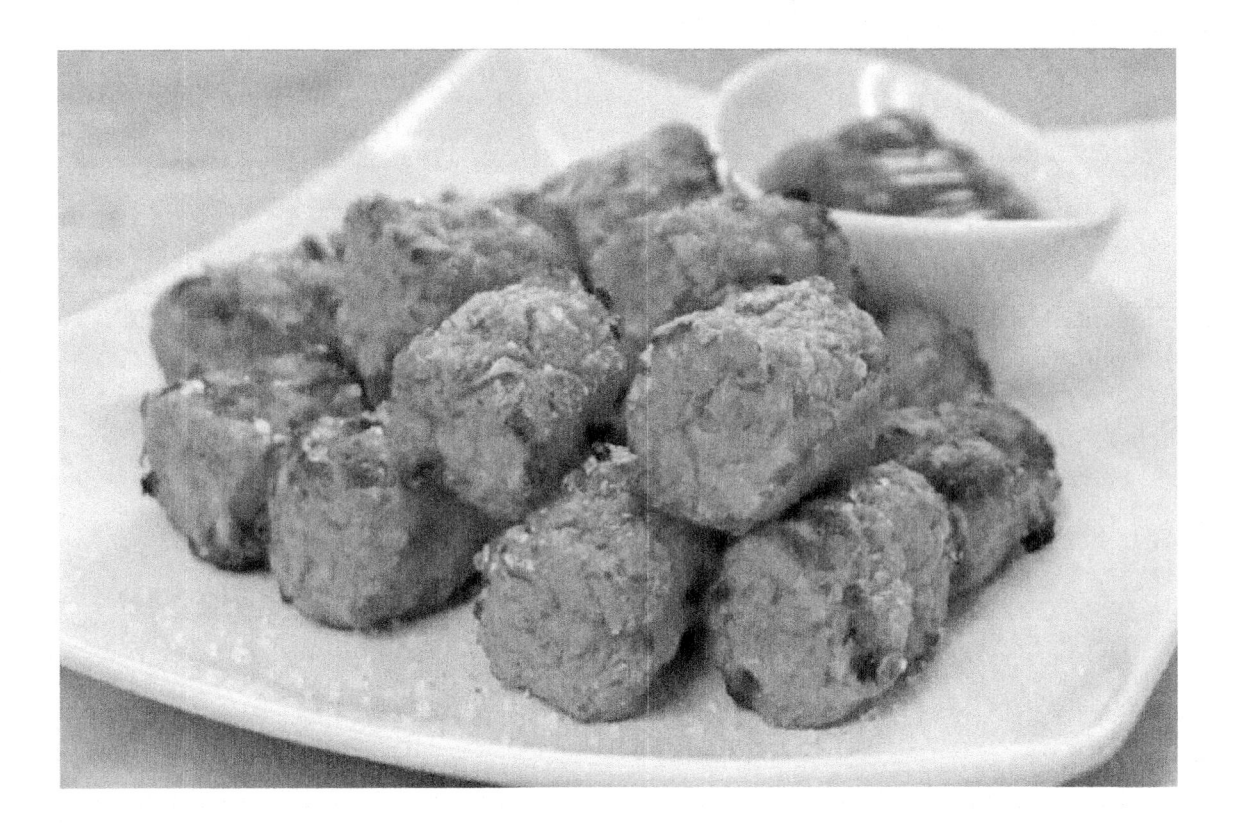

Crispy! Makes 2-4 servings.

Ingredients:

- 1 cup sweet potato mash
- 1/3 tablespoon chili powder
- 1/2 tablespoon paprika
- 1/4 tablespoon cayenne pepper
- 1/3 teaspoon garlic powder and parsley
- olive oil spray

Directions:

Mix sweet potato, chili powder, paprika, cayenne powder, garlic powder parsley.

With hands form into tater tots.

Lay out on plate.

Sprinkle both sides with spice mixture.

Lay aluminum foil in basket and place tots ½-inch apart.

Spray with oil.

Cook at 400 12-14 minutes.

Veggie Sliders

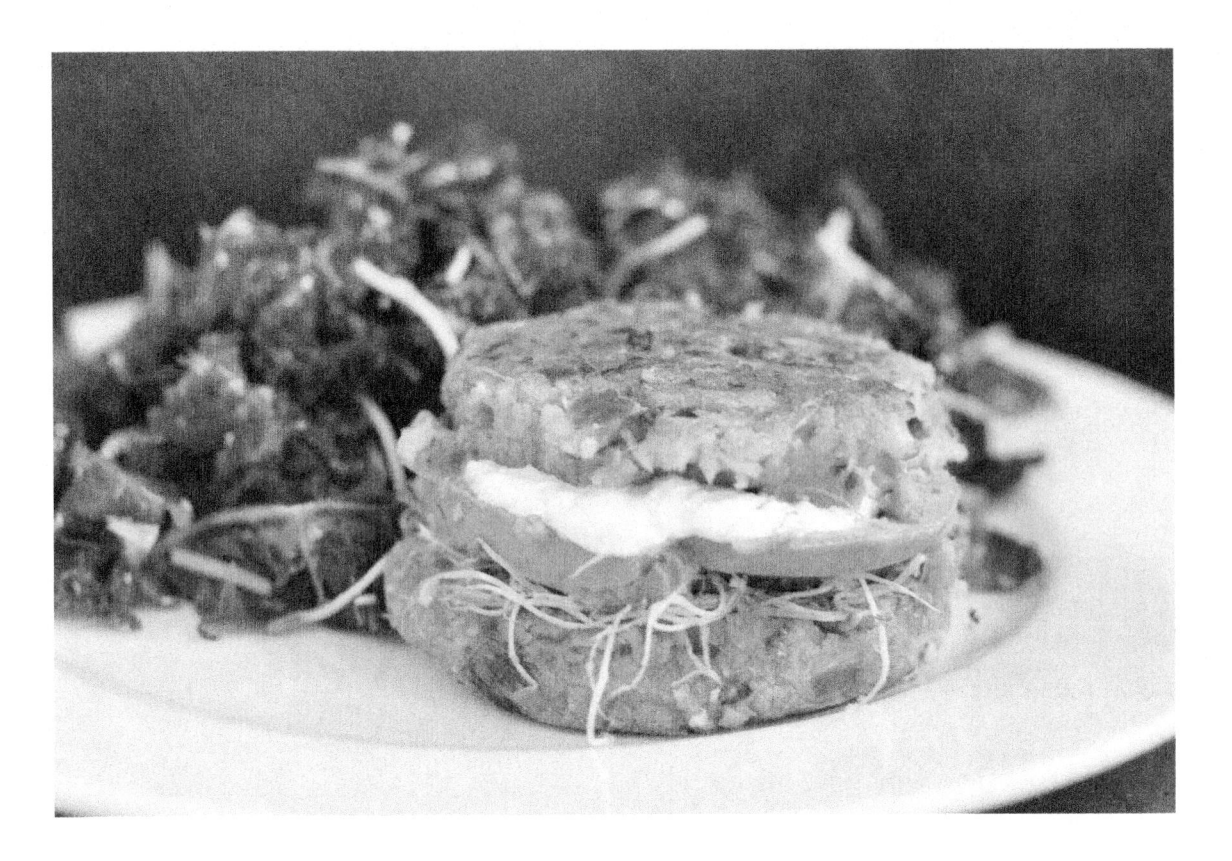

Try it with chicken! Makes 4 servings.

Ingredients:

- 2 cup garbanzo bean mash
- 2 eggs
- 1/3 cup shredded carrots
- ½ teaspoon garlic, minced
- 1 teaspoon onion, minced or grated
- 1/2 tablespoon ginger, minced
- 1/2 teaspoon brown sugar
- 1/4 teaspoon white pepper

Directions:

Mix garbanzo bean mash, eggs, shredded carrots, minced garlic, minced onion, minced ginger, brown sugar, white pepper, paprika.

Using hands form into 1-2 oz. patties.

Red Pepper and Feta Greek Gluten Free Pizza

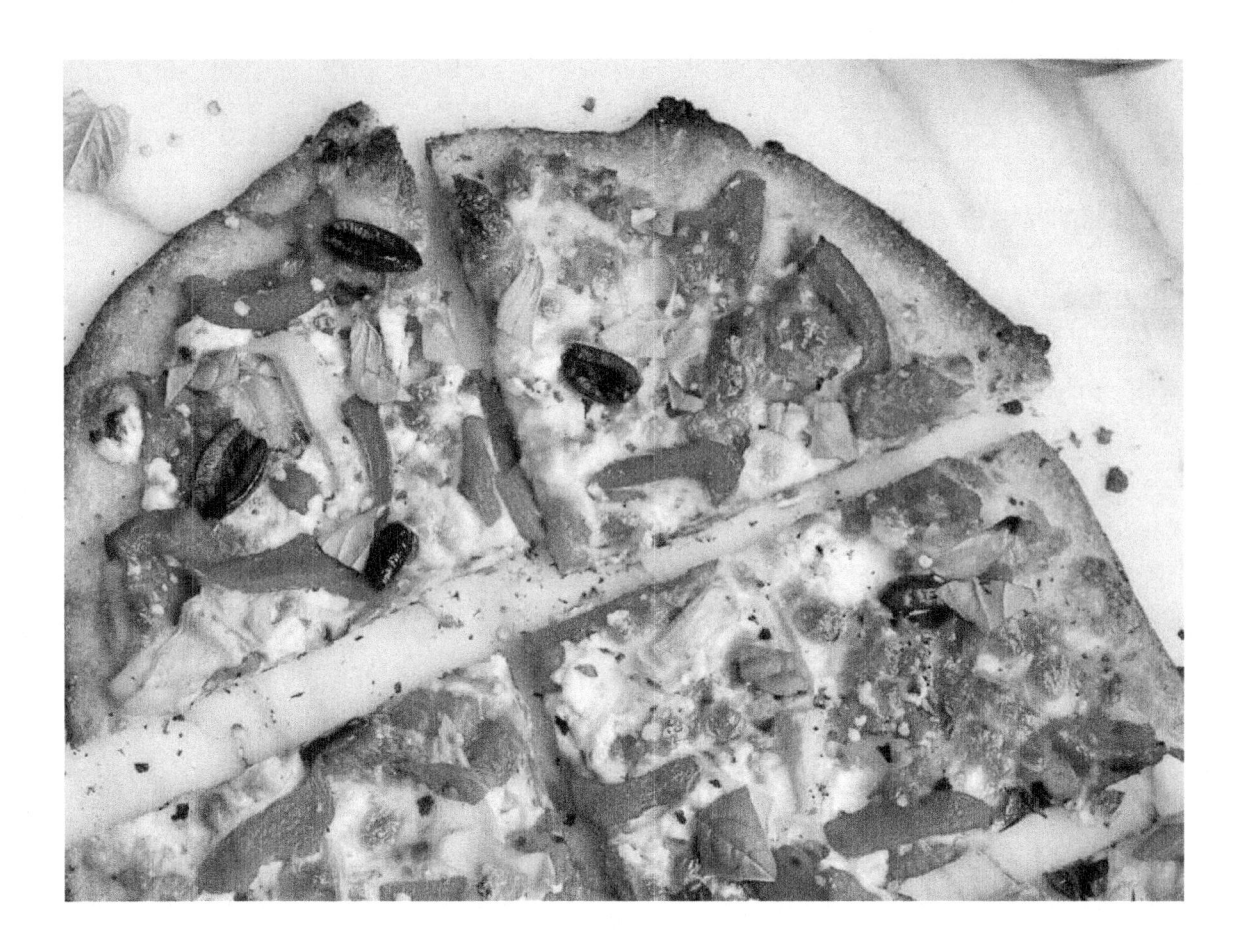

Try it with shredded chicken! Makes 1 personal pizza.

Ingredients:

- 1 gluten free personal pizza crust
- 1 tomato, chopped
- 1 red bell pepper, chopped
- 1/2 teaspoon Greek seasoning
- 1/2 teaspoon minced garlic
- 2 Tbsp crumbled feta cheese
- ¼ cup sliced mushrooms

Directions:

Preheat oven as directed on crust package and prepare baking sheet.

In food processor puree red bell pepper pieces and tomato pieces.

Spread evenly on pizza crust.

Top with seasoning, garlic, cheese, mushrooms.

BBQ Cauliflower Turkey Pizza

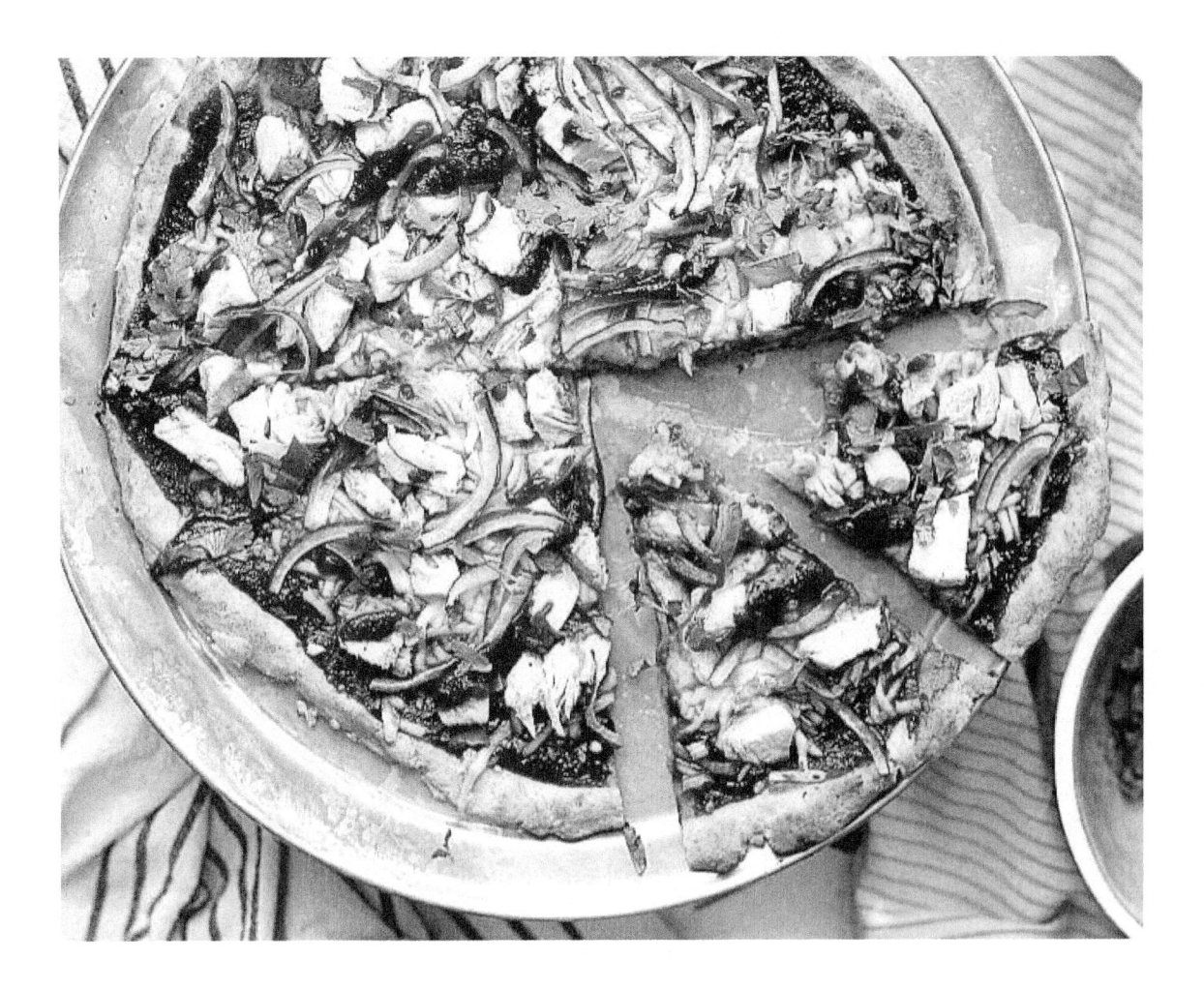

Try using different colored peppers! Makes 1 10-12-inch pizza.

Ingredients:

- 1/3 tsp sweet paprika
- ½ tsp garlic, minced
- 2 sweet red pepper, chopped- stems and seed removed
- 1 10-12-inch cauliflower pizza crust
- ¼ Favorite BBQ Sauce
- 2/3 cup ground turkey
- ½-1/3 cup shredded mozzarella cheese

Directions:

In blender or food processor add red pepper pieces, paprika, and minced garlic.

Puree or leave chunky-depends on thick you like your sauce.

Mix BBQ sauce into puree.

Spread evenly on cauliflower crust.

Top with shredded cheese, turkey.

Bake as directed on crust package.

2-Flour G.F. Pizza crust

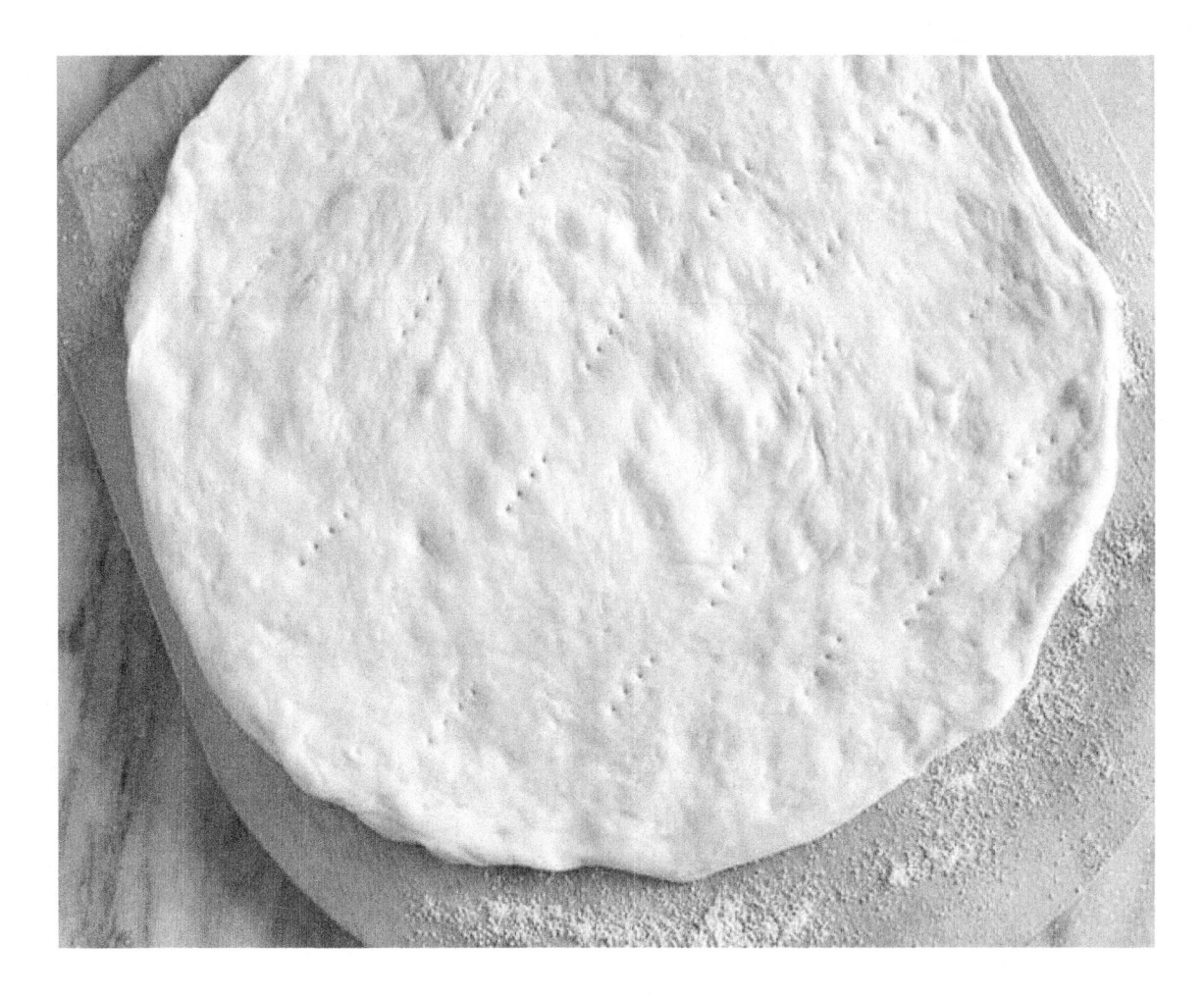

Great for all pizzas! Makes 1 12-14-inch pizza crust.

Ingredients:

- ¼ cup + 3 Tbsp coconut flour
- 1/2 cup + 3 Tbsp tapioca flour
- 3 Tbsp + ¼ cup olive oil
- 1/3 cup warm water
- 2 egg whites
- 1 egg yolk

Directions:

Preheat oven to 450 and prepare pizza stone.

Mix tapioca flour, coconut flour, and salt.

Pour in olive oil and water.

Add in egg whites and yolk and stir well.

Knead 1-3 minutes or until it forms a ball.

Dust a rolling pin with tapioca powder.

Roll out dough to a 12-14-inch crust.

Bake 12-15 minutes.

One Pot G.F. Andouille

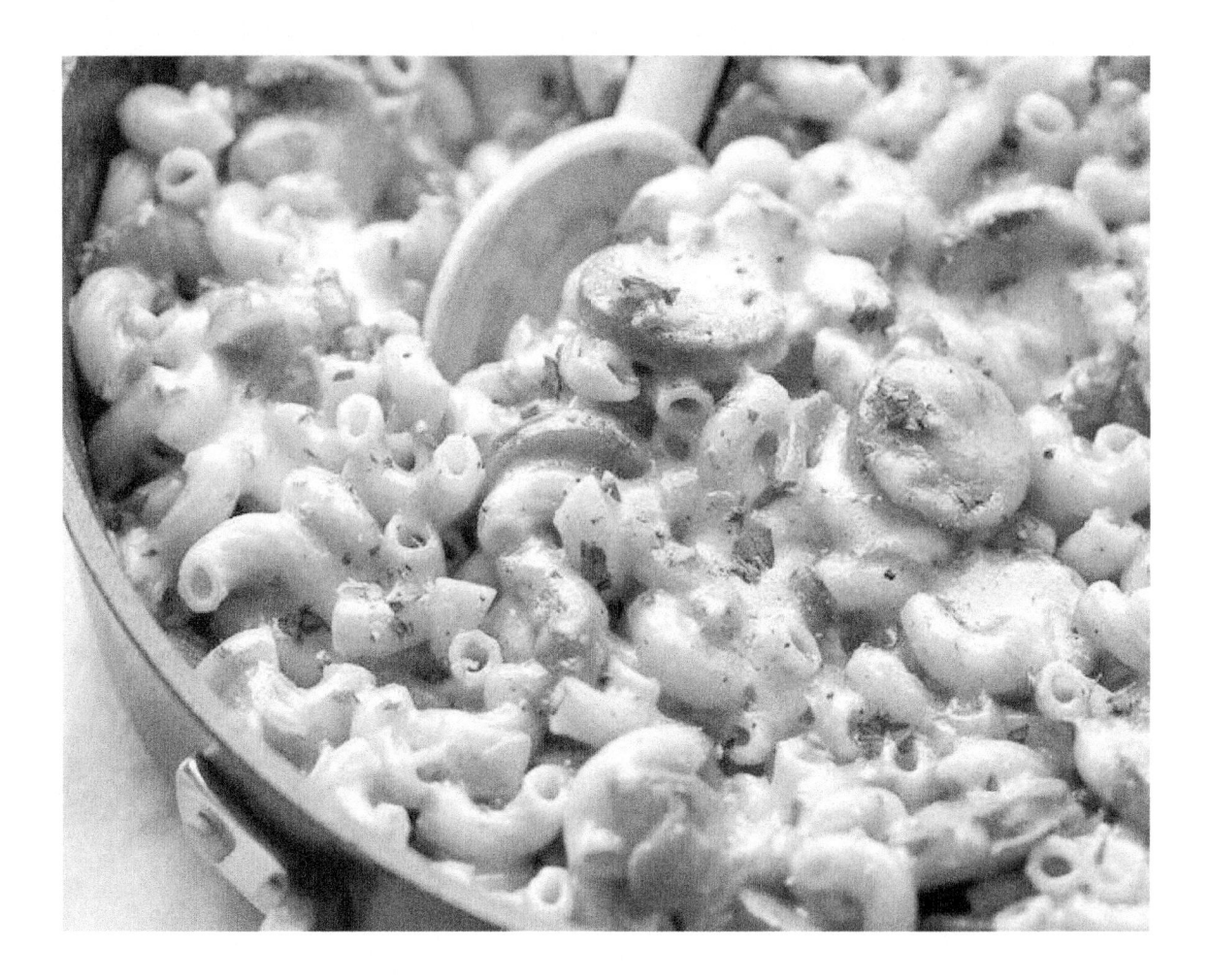

Do not forget the crunchy g.f. bread! Makes 3-4 servings.

Ingredients:

- 1/2 Tbsp olive oil
- 2-3cups diced andouille sausage
- 4 oz. uncooked gluten free spaghetti noodles
- 1 tsp salt free Italian seasoning
- 1/2 jar organic or all-natural spaghetti sauce (such as Ragu)
- 1 jar low sodium alfredo sauce
- ½ carton unsalted beef or chicken stock

Directions:

In pot bring water to a boil and add pasta.

Cook 8 minutes, drain, but do not rinse.

In separate pot add olive oil, sausage, spaghetti sauce, alfredo sauce, and stock. Stir well.

Bring to a boil; reduce heat, cover, and let simmer 18-20 minutes.

G.F. Apple Pie French Toast

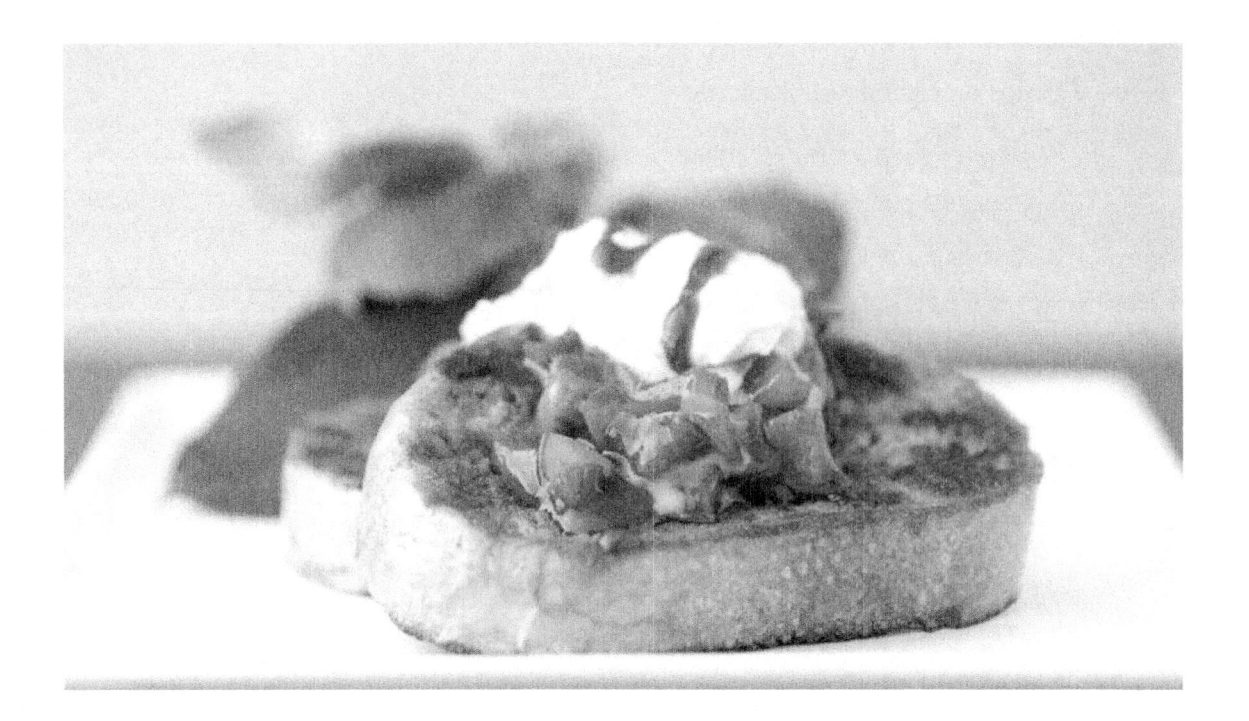

Add in extra cinnamon! Makes 1 serving.

Ingredients:

- 2-3 pieces gluten free white bread
- 1/2 teaspoon apple pie spice
- 2 eggs
- 1/3 cup unsweetened almond milk
- ½ Tbsp bread and butter extract

Directions:

Mix apple pie spice, unsweetened almond milk, eggs, extract.

Dip bread in mixture and place on griddle, cook 1 ½-2 minutes per side.

AND WASH IT DOWN WITH…

Gluten Dairy-Free Latte

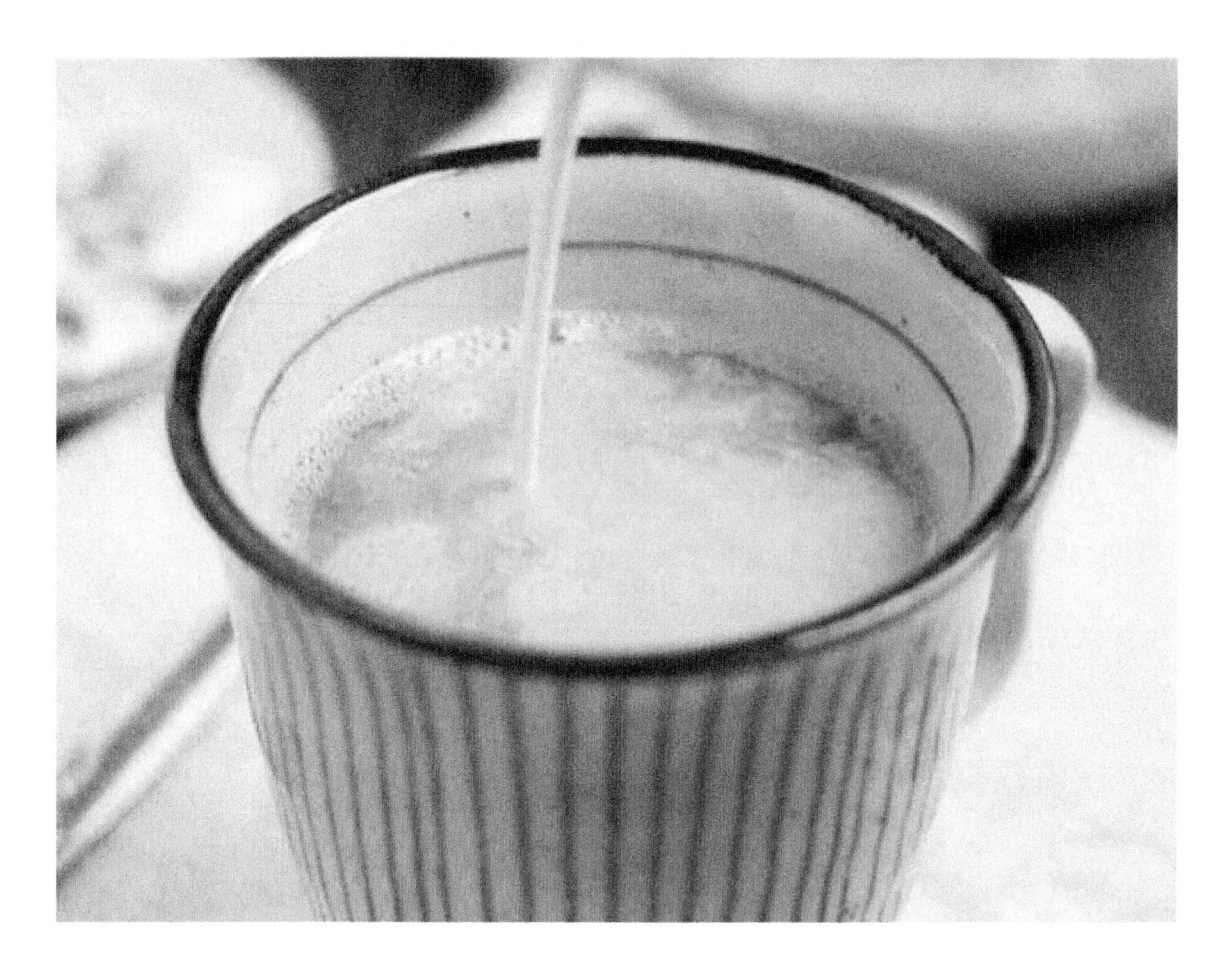

Why buy? Makes 1 serving.

Ingredients:

- 4-6 oz. serving strong coffee
- 3 tablespoons of cashews
- 2 teaspoons honey

Directions:

Blend coffee, cashews, and honey together starting low and working to high for about 40-45 seconds.

Gluten Free Treats

G.F. No-Bake Granola Bites

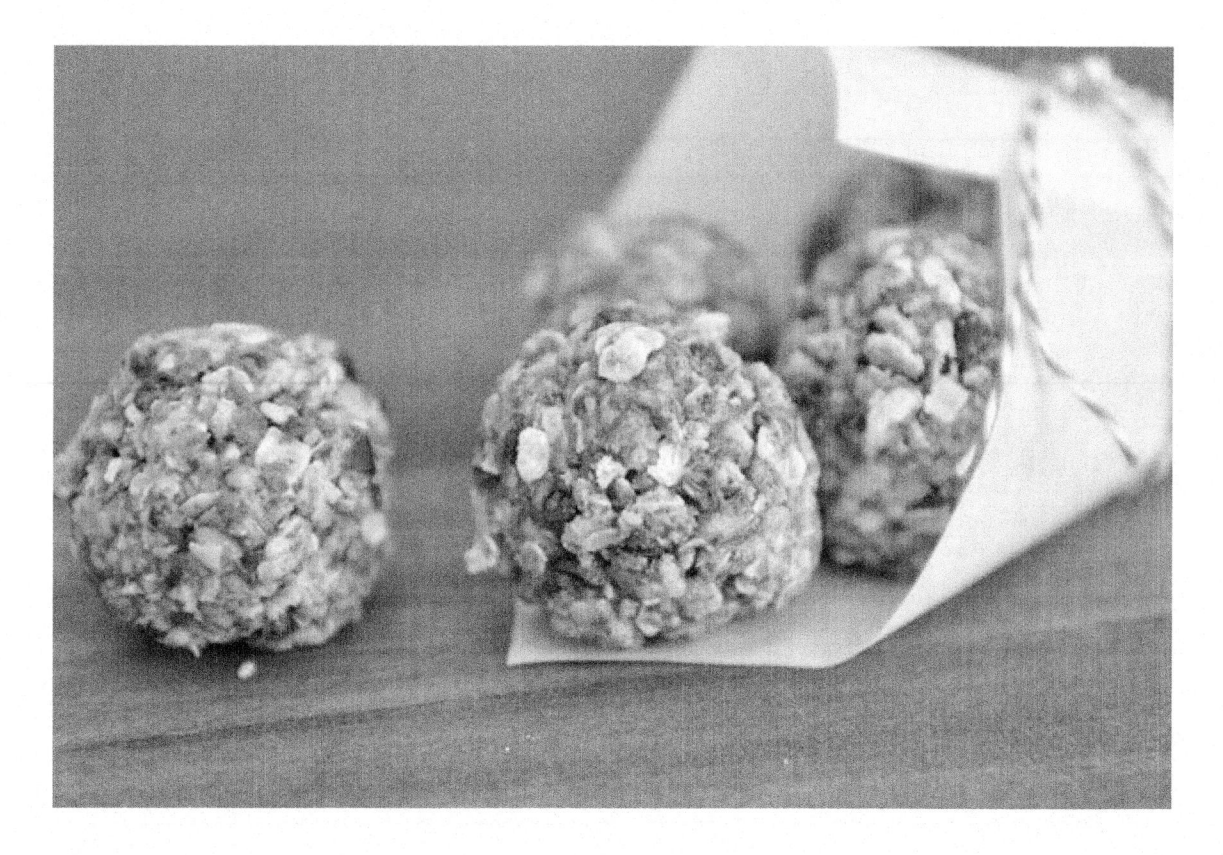

Good protein snacks! Makes approx. 9-12 servings.

Ingredients:

- 2 tablespoon organic honey
- 3/4 cup g.f peanut butter
- ½ tsp butter nut flavored extract
- 1 Tbsp brown sugar
- 1 bag flavored g.f. cereal such as Chex Granola Mixed Berry Almond
- 1/3 cup chocolate chips
- 1/3 cup peanut butter chips

Directions:

Line baking tray with parchment.

In a bowl mix together cereal, chocolate chips, and peanut butter chips.

In saucepan over medium high heat add and stir continuously: honey, peanut butter, extract.

With spoon or ice cream scoop, lay out granola bites 2-inches apart then chill in refrigerator 30 minutes.

Bananas and Berries

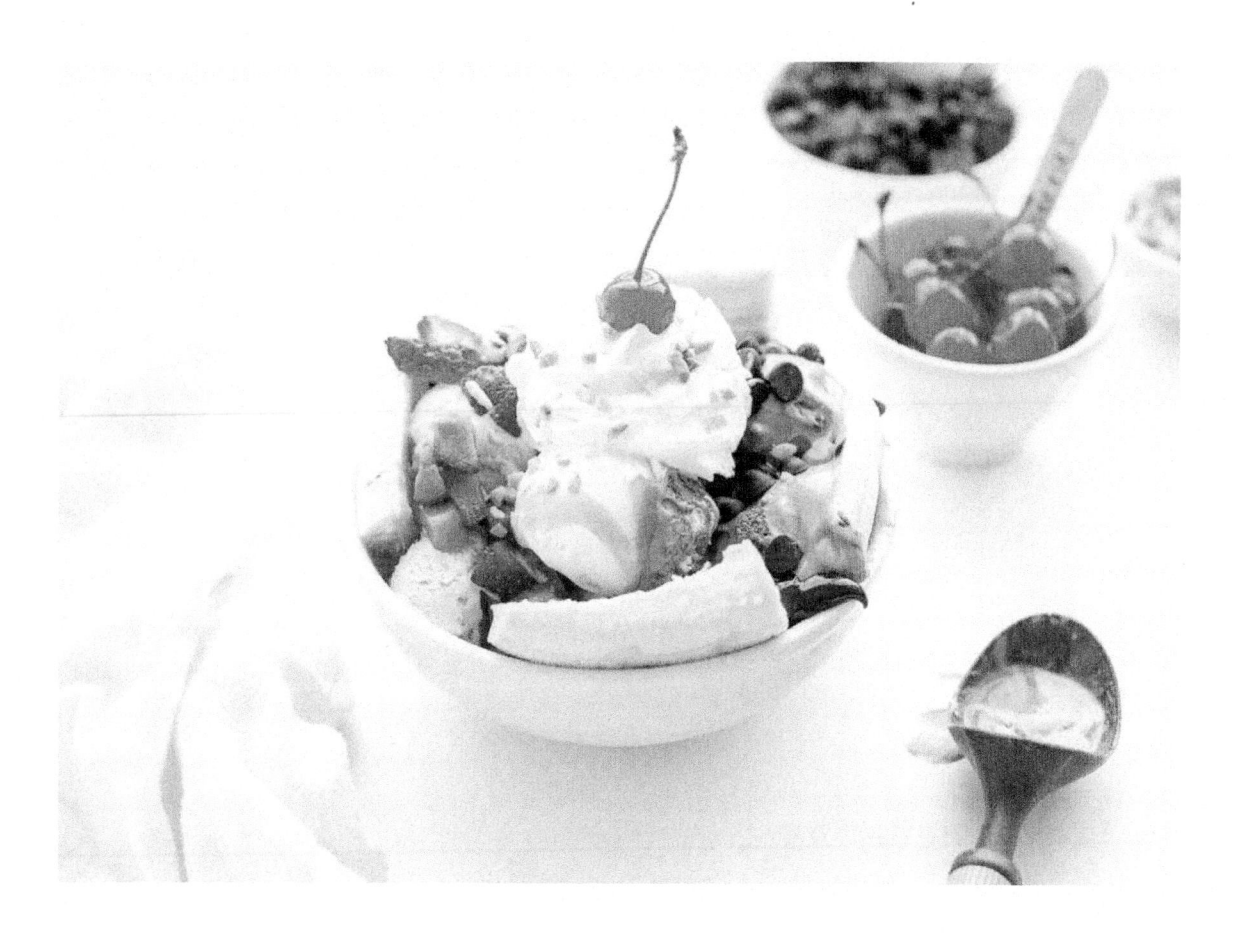

Delicious! Makes 2 servings.

Ingredients:

- 1/3 cup chopped strawberries
- Maple syrup
- Chocolate syrup
- 1 banana, halved
- 3 cup whipped cream or Neapolitan ice cream

Directions:

Preheat oven to 400 and line baking tray with parchment paper.

Layout strawberries on tray, drizzle with maple syrup, bake 18-22 minutes.

Meanwhile toasted coconut and walnuts in skillet set over med.-low heat.

Place bananas horizontally and top with whipped cream or ice cream.

Top with strawberries and syrup.

Easy Gluten Free Nutella Brownies

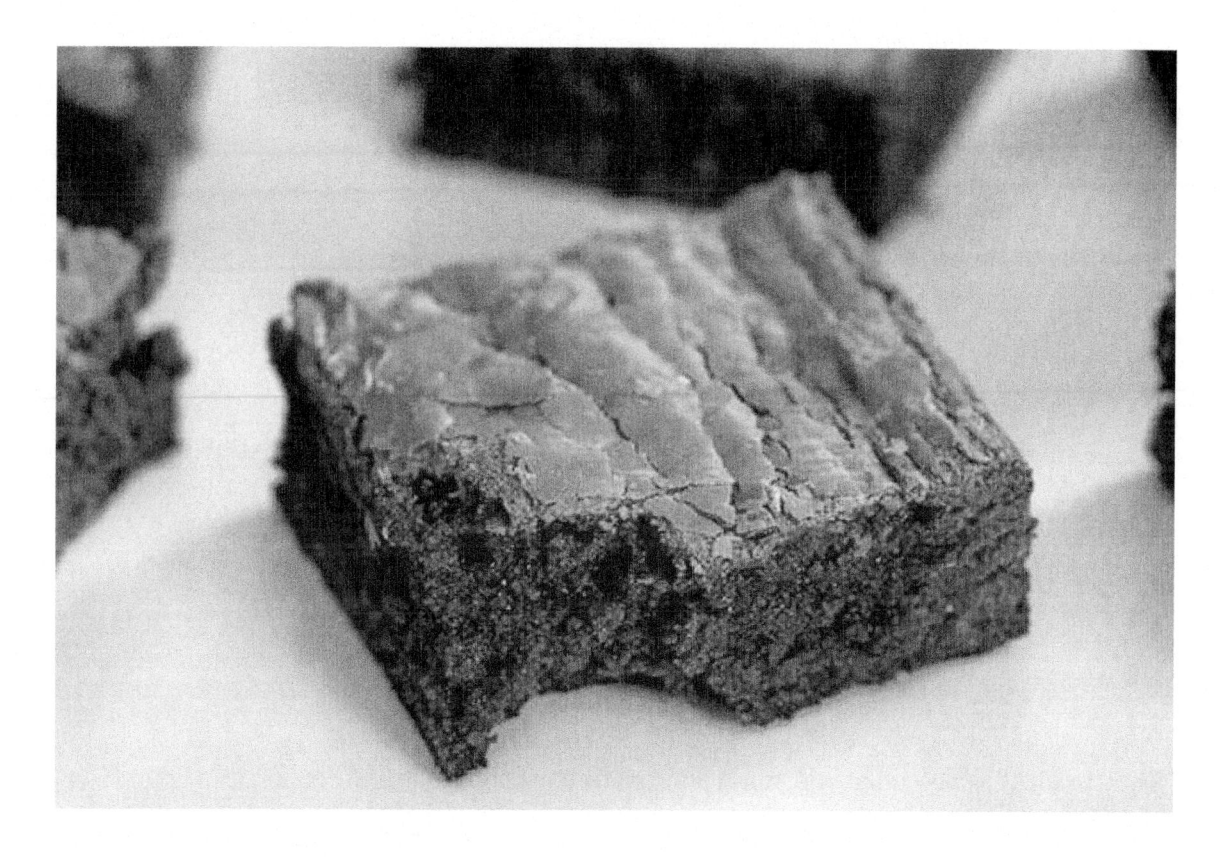

Great for brownies! Makes approx. 1 – 1 ½ cups.

Ingredients:

- 1 cup almond flour
- 1 1/2 tablespoon unsweetened cacao powder or blend carob pieces till a powder
- 1 Tbsp organic honey, agave, or sugar-free maple syrup (optional)
- 2 Tbsp chocolate-hazelnut spread (such as Nutella)
- 2 eggs

Directions:

Mix almond flour; cacao powder or carob powder; honey, agave, or syrup; chocolate-hazelnut spread; eggs.

Pour into 8x8 pan.

Bake 20-25 minutes.

When pouring, if too thick add small amount of sunflower butter or coconut oil.

Peanut Butter Brownies

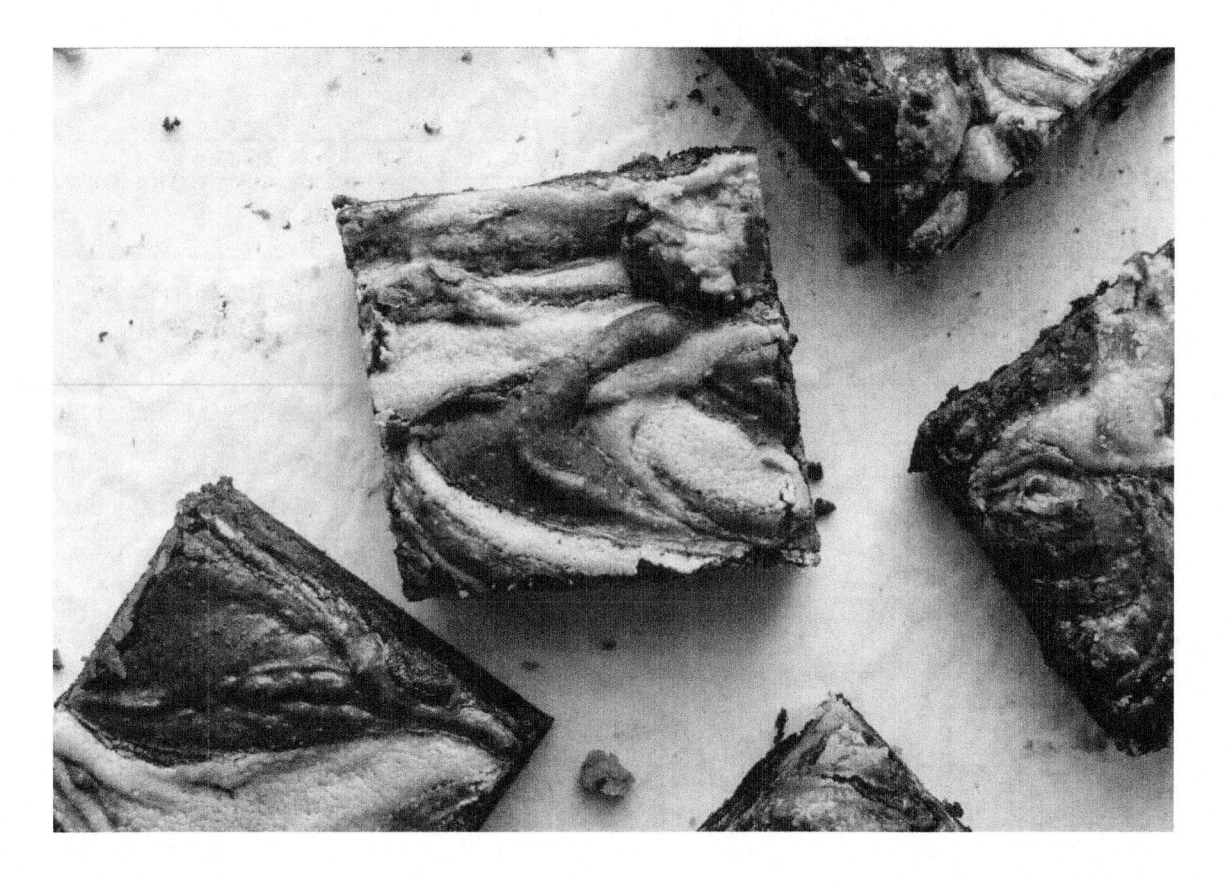

Guilt free deliciousness! Makes 9 servings.

Ingredients:

- 1/3 cup coconut oil, melted
- 4 heaping tablespoons cocoa powder
- 2 oz unsweetened bakers' chocolate
- 2/3 cup honey or agave
- 2 large eggs, room temperature
- 1 teaspoon vanilla
- 1/4 cup coconut flour
- 1 cup natural or organic peanut butter, melted
- 1 package peanut butter chips

Directions:

Preheat oven to 350 and prepare a 9x9 dish by lining it with parchment paper.

In saucepan over medium heat melt coconut oil, cocoa powder, and unsweetened Bakers' chocolate. Stirring until there are no lumps.

Add in, honey, eggs, vanilla, coconut flour, melted peanut butter, beating well after each addition:

Mix in peanut butter chips.

Pour into 9x9 pan and bake 20-25 minutes, store in airtight container in refrigerator.

G.F. Mini Mallow Toffee Brownies

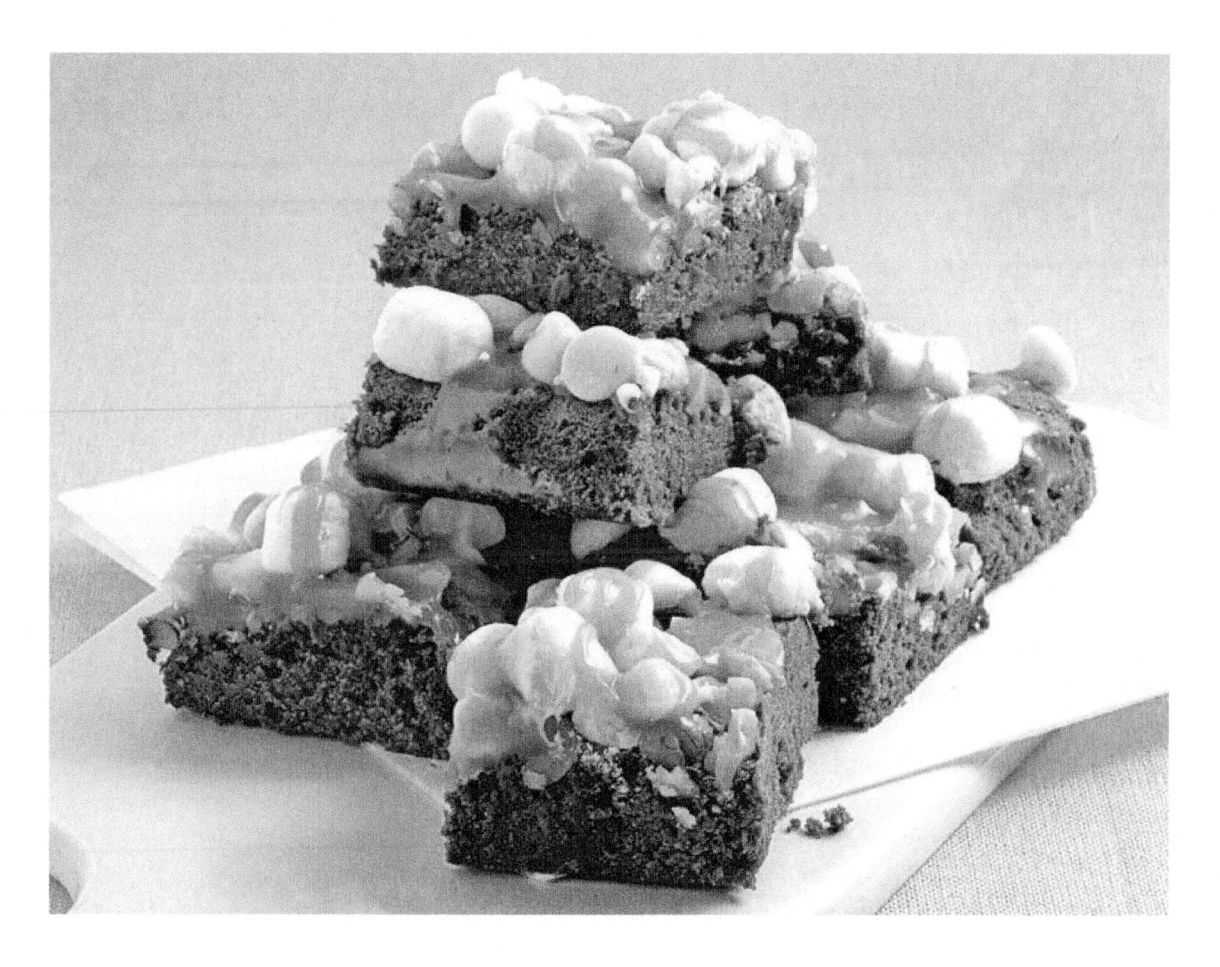

Mint chips are good too! Makes 8-10 servings.

Ingredients:

- 2 Tbsp coconut oil, melted
- 2 ½ tablespoons cocoa powder
- 2 oz unsweetened bakers' chocolate
- 2/3 Tbsp honey or agave
- 2 large eggs, room temperature
- 1/2 teaspoon vanilla extract
- 1/4 cup almond flour
- 1 cup mini marshmallows
- 6 oz. package organic peanut butter chips

Directions:

Preheat oven to 350 and prepare a 9x9 dish by lining it with parchment paper.

In saucepan over medium heat melt coconut oil, cocoa powder, and unsweetened Bakers' chocolate. Stirring until there are no lumps.

Add in beating well after each addition: honey, eggs, vanilla, coconut flour, mint extract, mini marshmallows, toffee chips.

Pour into 9x9 pan and bake 23-28 minutes, store in airtight container in refrigerator.

G.F. Chocolate Bread

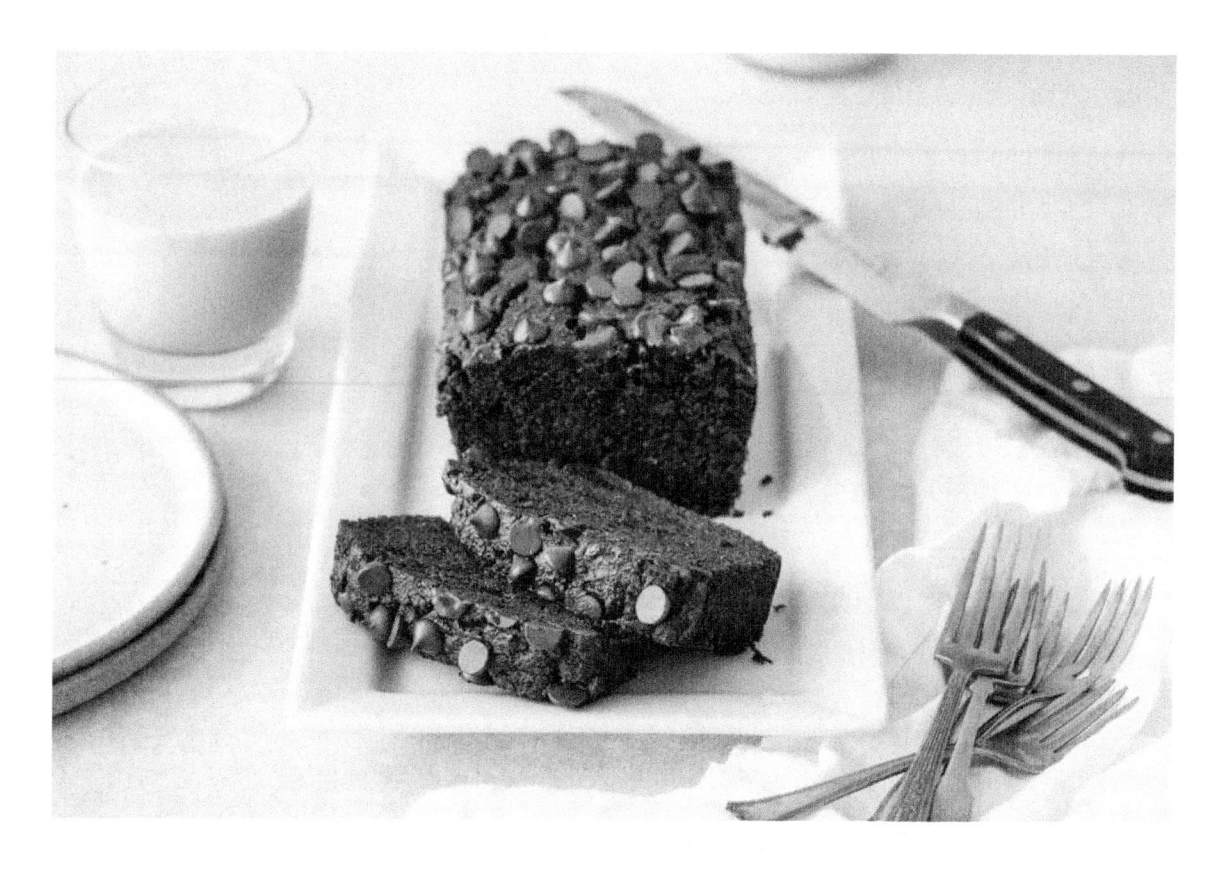

Makes a great "just because" gift! Makes approx. 10 slices.

Ingredients:

- 3/4 cup beets
- ¾ cup almond flour
- 1/3 cup coconut flour
- 1/4 cup maple syrup
- 1/3 cup cocoa powder
- 1/3 cup coconut milk
- 3 egg whites
- 1 egg yolk
- 1 teaspoon vanilla extract
- 1 package dark chocolate chips
- 1/3 teaspoon baking soda

Directions:

Preheat oven to 350 and line loaf pan with parchment paper.

Microwave beets 4-5 minutes then set aside.

Whisk together almond coconut flour, cocoa powder, baking powder.

Blend until smooth: coconut milk, eggs, yolk, syrup, vanilla extract, beets.

Pour liquid ingredients into dry and stir. Pour into loaf pan and bake 45-55 minutes.

Seal leftovers in airtight container in refrigerator will keep 1 week.

Author's Afterthoughts

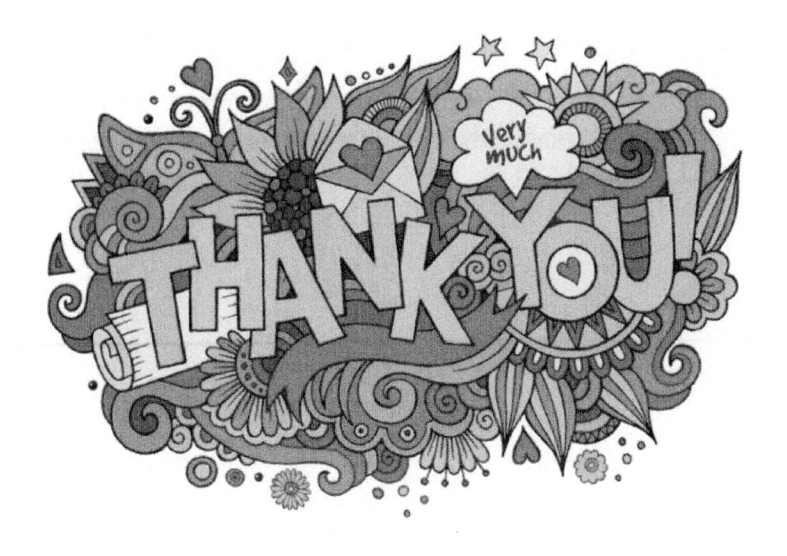

Thanks ever so much to each of my cherished readers for investing the time to read this book!

I know you could have picked from many other books, but you chose this one. So, a big thanks for reading all the way to the end. If you enjoyed this book or received value from it, I'd like to ask you for a favor. Please take a few minutes to **post an honest and heartfelt review on** *Amazon.com.* Your support does make a difference and helps to benefit other people.

Thanks!

Julia Chiles

Printed in Great Britain
by Amazon